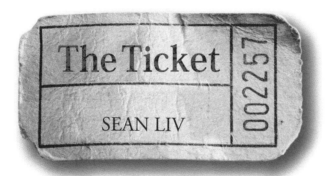

The Ticket

SEAN LIV

002257

Unite your body, mind and spirit for a powerful life.

Published by Liv Publishing

Visit us at www.seanliv.com
or www.thetickettochange.com

Cover designed by: Seven Ink Design Ltd.
Edited by: Samantha Garner
Photography by: Chantal Milaine Photography
Cover Portrait by: Heather Mudry at Movi Photography

Library and Archives Canada Cataloguing in Publication

Liv, Sean
    The ticket : unite your body, mind and spirit for a powerful life / Sean
Liv.

Includes index.
ISBN 978-0-9813986-0-0

    1. Weight loss--Psychological aspects. 2. Self-actualization (Psychology).
3. Change (Psychology). 4. Health behavior. I. Title.

RM222.2.L59 2010   613.2'5   C2010-903294-2

Printed by: Petro-Tech Printing Ltd.
          Calgary, AB
Published and distributed in Canada by:
Sean Liv Productions INC.

Important: The author of this book is not responsible for any injuries incurred, and strongly advises the advice of a physician before starting any program. The intent of the author of this book is to offer information of a general intent to help you in your quest for finding the power within yourself, Body, Mind, and Spirit. In the event you use any of the information in this book for yourself, which is your constitutional right, the author and publisher assume no responsibility for your actions.

To Rob, my husband, my best friend
Thank you for all your support as I continue to
walk the path of my dreams.

To Hannah, my inspiration
You are my courage, my strength
and my sidekick!

I love you both

....

And to you,
The fearless leader in your own life.

TABLE OF CONTENTS

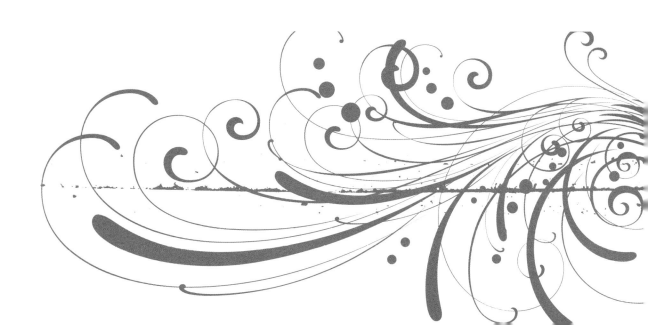

Precautions: Before you Begin

Before beginning any exercise program, consult your doctor to review any potential health risks that may be present. Visiting your doctor is especially important if you have had a recent injury, illness or are undergoing rehabilitation treatment. If you experience dizziness, nausea, excessive shortness of breath, or chest pain, stop the activity and let your doctor know. Be sure to check all exercise equipment and locations to make sure they're safe and strong.

ACKNOWLEDGMENTS

This book/program would not have been possible without the incredible people who have been placed upon my path to make it happen.

Thank you to all of my clients. You embarked upon a fearless journey by not only listening to my guidance but to your inner strength and determination. Thank you for allowing this program to evolve into what it is.

My father, Bill, my biggest fan. I continue to be inspired by your nine years of sobriety. Your courage and inner strength to change is what true commitment and determination is about. Thank you for your love and support.

My mother, Mary. Thank you for your endless hours of editing. You are my mother, a sister and my friend. Thank you for our endless conversations together as we journey through the beautiful creation of life.

My wonderful husband, Rob. My confidant, my best friend. I am the luckiest woman to be married to a man who has supported me throughout this entire journey. Thank you for your gentleness, your understanding and believing in my dreams. I am honoured to be sharing my life with such an incredible man.

My daughter Hannah. You are my inspiration, my courage, and my strength. Without you this book would not exist. You are the reason for this. I love you!

Chantal, my photographer. Your passion and spirit inspires me. Thank you for your time and talent with the photography throughout this book.

Samantha, my editor. You transformed the pages upon pages of my thoughts into what it is now. You embarked upon this project with dedication and pride and I will always be so grateful for you and your talent.

Jen, my designer, your talent is undeniable. Your keen eye and your creativity have made this bigger then I could have imagined. Your heart and soul are present throughout.

My friend Carol. Thank You for your help and advice.

Diane, my healer. You are light. You are love. You are an angel. You have truly helped me heal into the spirit in which I am today. Thank you for giving me the healing energy from the divine.

My Angels and Spirit. Thank you for the wonderful miracle of life itself. Thank you for your guidance and lighting the way for the creation of this book. Thank you for the joys, the sorrows and the amazing transformation one receives when they discover their ultimate power.

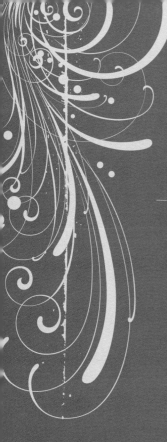

Be Courage, where there is Courage there is Strength and where there is Strength there is POWER

Introduction

CHAPTER ONE: How it Began

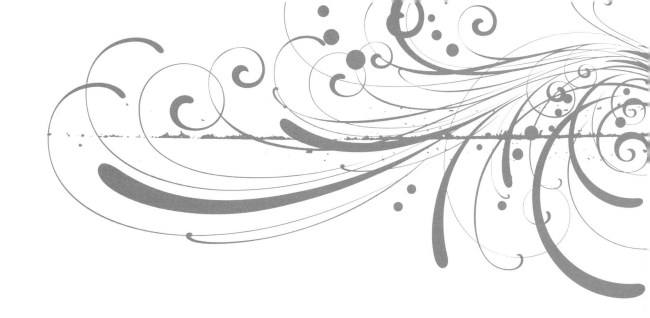

Chapter One
HOW IT BEGAN

"Dreams are the touchstones of our characters."

Henry David Thoreau

HOW IT BEGAN

My Own Journey

My childhood was a challenging one, coming from a family with an alcoholic father and a submissive mother. Growing up, I didn't learn how to stand up for myself. I didn't have a strong voice. I dropped out of high school and fell into drugs and minor criminal activity. I found myself in an abusive relationship on a path of hardship, abuse, poor discipline and negativity.

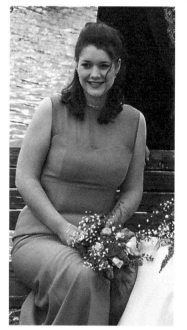

20lbs lost with a secret life of drugs, abuse and fear.

As I matured, I began a career that I enjoyed, in management and training. The development I gained from this career allowed me to find strength and courage to leave my abusive relationship. It was a huge step in my life, but I was left alone with almost nothing to my name and a self-esteem that was hanging by a thread. My career was all that kept me going, but I needed skills and knowledge. I needed answers about my life.

I began to focus on building my career, working my way up the corporate ladder. I met and married a wonderful man and became pregnant with our daughter. I was finishing up my year on maternity leave, when my dream job within the company came up. It was what I had spent seven years preparing myself for. And I didn't get it.

I was at one of my lowest of lows. I had worked so hard, despite my rough start in life, and I felt cheated out of something that could have changed my life. The fact that I was still carrying the extra weight from my pregnancy made me feel even worse. I found it hard to get out of bed in the morning. I was in a state of depression. I had no self-esteem, no self-worth, no passion or enthusiasm for life.

I merely existed.

I had been there many times before. I had many hours of talk therapy under my belt and had read loads of self-help books. The difference was, this time I just did not want to share all my thoughts and emotions with a stranger all over again.

This was the turning point in my life. I was tired of depression, tired of the negative self-talk and tired of the darkness that surrounded my life. For some reason, this time was about me. All the promises I'd made to myself over the years finally clicked. I knew I had to make major changes in my life in order to change my past. A sentence popped into my head. It was, "If you can't trust yourself, then who can you trust?" This resonated hugely with me. Throughout my entire life, there was no one who had not hurt me in some way and, of course, I include myself in that. For that reason finding and discovering trust within myself was an incredible, impossible thing.

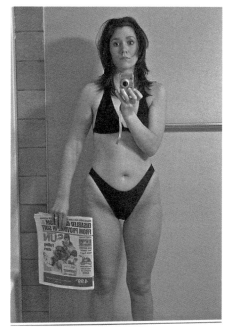

Who am I?

It All Started With a Bikini

It was January 2nd when I made the commitment to finally work towards one of my dreams. This dream was to wear a bikini. I went through a period in my life from the age of 12 to 20 when my weight reached an all time high of just over 200 pounds. I managed to lose some of the weight but couldn't get past my plateau. I had tried the diets, the pills and the powders but none of them seemed to work. None of them allow you to enter inside yourself to see the real reason for the weight. They are all fixated upon the number on a scale or a certain size of pants. They don't go further than a list of ingredients on a label.

liv

There I was, with all of my previous failed attempts and a bottom of the barrel self-esteem. I had nothing but a vision of completely changing my body and wearing a bikini.

So I began on my journey. My "before" picture was the first thing I did, for my challenge of self discovery. Completely embarrassed of my body, not even allowing my husband to take the picture, I stood in front of the mirror in a bathing suit, holding a paper to mark the day.

Next was finding the body of my dreams. Of course, I had lots of fitness magazines lying around so it wasn't hard to flip through and find the vision I was searching for. I cut the head off of the model and it became the image of my journey. I used it as the cover image of an inspiration book I created for my personal challenge.

Next, I made a contract to myself. I typed a few words on the computer, dated it, printed it and signed it. This was the next page of my inspiration book.

My intentions page came next. This is where I set a few intentions, not necessarily as goals, but as promises to myself. Things like *I will take it one step at a time. I will do my best every day to love myself as I am.*

After that, I created a page containing affirmations I felt would help me heal my past. These affirmations were words and phrases that I came up with to help me start, but to also give myself the momentum to keep going.

The next page was my measurement page, where I had my starting weight and my physical measurements. I used this page to track my measurements every four weeks. From there I created a soundtrack for the journey, my all-time faves. This helped me stay motivated and inspired during my workouts.

I created an exercise and nutrition plan. I took it day by day, from my workouts, to my meals, to the affirmations and so forth. As the days went by, I started to celebrate the empowerment I was beginning to feel. I started to learn everything that I needed to know to make the right food and exercise choices. This was a whole learning process for me, as I had no previous exercise or nutrition experience. But I stuck to it and it became part of my routine and my life.

Transforming More Than My Body

I was off. I had completed all of my workouts and, yes, my eating choices were in line with the program. At the end of the week, I received a comment from my husband that will always stay with me. I was sitting on the living room floor, having a lazy Saturday evening, unconcerned about how I looked - and my husband told me that I looked hot. From this comment, I gained even more momentum to continue.

When I started this journey it was a complete low in my life and the only person who knew that I was doing this challenge was me. I never shared it with a soul. This was a commitment that I had made for myself to myself. This was something that I was going to do on my own.

In order to keep myself on track, I decided to give myself a weekly gift. My first week's gift was a pair of pajamas, and I continued to reward myself week after week. Sometimes it was just a new colour of nail polish, other times is was more, like a new pair of shoes. It did wonders for my motivation and even made me feel a little pampered!

The first couple of weeks of my journey were the hardest - physically, mentally and emotionally. Everything was so new. I was holding my book while exercising to check my form, I was trying new recipes and fitting in my basement workouts while still doing all of my other household tasks. It was nuts, but there was something deep within me that kept me going. My spirit wanted to evolve. She wanted to become alive, she wanted to become free.

In my third week I started to see some changes within my body. My spirit was growing and I was feeling incredible. At about the four week mark, I was getting out of bed before my entire family to keep my appointment with myself in my basement. I loved it. It was my time, my theme songs, my power words. I was able to step out of the roles I was playing in life and just be. I was able to see who was in me, what she liked to do, where she wanted to go, and what she was really like.

After that, every morning was like Christmas. My physique was changing, my emotions were healing and my spirit began to be seen. My thoughts, my music and my power words helped me continue the challenge.

I remember my last cardio workout like it was yesterday. I was on my elliptical completing day 84 when a feeling of complete emotion came over me, I finally completed something in my life, for me. I did it for no one else. Not even my husband knew about my challenge and my dreams until he started to notice the changes. The transformation of myself ultimately began the journey to know and heal my whole self - mind, body and spirit. I finally loved the person looking back at me in the mirror.

The Dream of a Lifetime

After four weeks into this mini journey, I knew I wanted to do this for a living. I wanted to become a personal trainer. It became not just a physical goal, but, a spiritual and mental goal. This became another challenge for me, as I was carrying around a lot of negative past energy about school. My high school years weren't the greatest and, in fact, I never graduated. So, when applying into college, I not only had to write a pre-exam and get at least 65% to pass, but I also had to face old wounds of being a high school drop out.

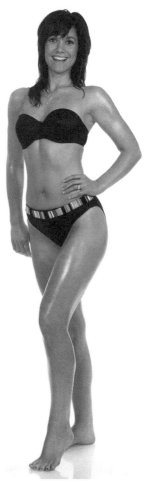

School started in September and it was a long, long wait. As with my physical challenge, I never told a soul about my decision. It was something that I wanted deeply, that was mine. I was still using the same principles of positive thoughts, power words, music and exercise. The difference is that now I was pursuing my dream of going to college. All my thoughts shifted towards this.

On August 18, I received a call from the college saying that I was accepted and I needed to drop off the tuition. I was thrilled, but also nervous. This was my dream. I was going to go to college, but the hurdle was the tuition fee. I never told my husband that I had applied for college, I didn't tell a soul. All I have ever had was faith and trust with something higher than myself, whatever name you want to give it. I needed a miracle.

So we were all in the bathroom with my daughter in the tub. I took a deep breath and said, "Honey, I did something." "What did you do?" He replied nervously, as if I messed something up with our contracting business that I managed.
I blurted it out - "I applied to college and I was accepted."

I held my breath. This was the turning point to make my dream a reality. I didn't know what he was going to say, or how he would react. I had never thought about that side of it.

He looked at our daughter in the tub and said to her, "Your mommy did good! She's going to college!"

I was finally achieving a dream of going to college that I never thought was possible. My teenage years and early 20s were filled with drugs, addictions and abuse. My confidence and self worth were completely gone. This was amazing. I remember walking down the halls of the college embracing that I was finally a college student. All of the small details seemed to work themselves out and I was able to pursue my dream even with all I had to be responsible for in my life.

I continued with my motivation, every morning, with myself and my music. My time, dreams, words and my spirit continuing to evolve. The dream of my business, the dream of graduating college with my daughter watching and the belief in spirit, that this was my path - all these dreams made this possible. My graduation day came and went, and it was an amazing trip.

Find the Power of Your Dreams
From there I created a personal training company where I wanted to test what I

had discovered with myself, and to help others find their motivation and passion for life. I was very successful and met hundreds of amazing people through my outdoor boot camps, personal training clients, nutritional consulting, program designs, as well as workshops and grocery store tours.

It was a real eye opener. I discovered the hard way that most people are only looking for the quick fixes, the magic pills or powders and are afraid to look within to discover the REAL Motivation. Sure, I was able to offer inspiration and motivation, but to really change your life, to really become fearless and tackle your dreams, only you can do it. The power of your dreams lies within you, and until you tap into your spirit to ignite these powers they will remain dormant.

I believe that we all have so much potential within us, that is just waiting to be discovered. I never dreamed that I would be a personal trainer, a published author, or even the creator of this program. I was a high school dropout, a former drug addict recovering from a past abusive relationship. My self-esteem and confidence was zero. Going from the bottom to where I am now, all on my own, through transforming my mind, body and spirit is truly amazing. There is something magical when we allow ourselves to face our demons to heal our past, gain strength in the present and have faith and trust for the future. Even with all of my talk therapy over the years nothing compares to taking your life in your own hands. You, connecting to a power inside yourself that is your own compass, your map, your guide. This life that you are living is yours to live, and no one else can fulfill what is in you. No one else can discover your own truth, your own strength and ultimately your own purpose.

Allow your present to dictate your future. Allow your past to be healed. Allow your spirit to be ignited to light your way. Be power, be passion, be freedom, be love, be voice, be wisdom, be purpose.

Namaste,
Sean Liv

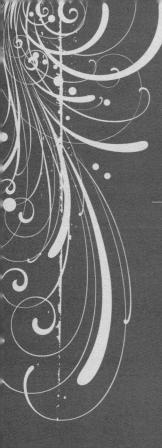

Be Pride, where there is Pride there is Passion and where there is Passion there is CREATION

Mind

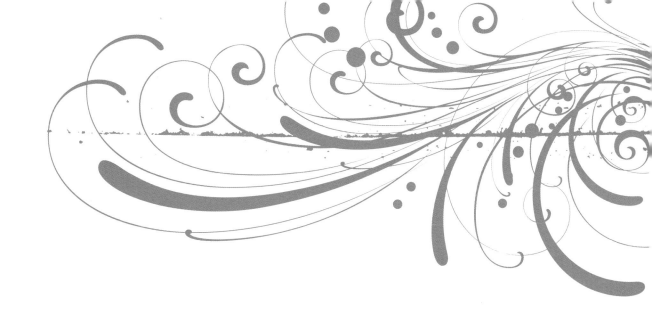

Chapter Two
REAL MOTIVATION

"Life takes on meaning when you become motivated.
Set goals and charge after them in
an unstoppable manner."

Les Brown

REAL MOTIVATION

It's amazing how many people's dreams go by without a second thought. It's as if we believe that our dreams can't come true, or that it could never happen to us.

What happened to the childlike wonder within all of us that allows us to dream? I'm talking about dreaming of what you truly want in life, living a life knowing and believing in endless possibilities: your perfect profession; building your dream house; vacationing all around the world; writing a novel; watching your seeds grow in the garden; cooking for your family and friends; designing a clothing line or maybe even performing on stage with a band!

What happened to the dreaming? What happened to believing in the future? Let's see if we can get it back for just a few minutes.

Take some time to let your mind wander and imagine. Imagine it's the first day of your ideal life. You wake up in the morning, get out of bed and stretch your arms in the air. You look around and realize you are finally living in your dream house. What does it look like? Is it small and cozy or spacious and grand?

Imagine yourself getting ready for your morning shower. You catch a glimpse of yourself in the mirror and your stature is strong, your shoulders are held back with pride, your eyes are as clear as can be.

As you start your day, who is there to greet you? Is it your children? Your spouse or partner? Maybe it's a loving pet. Imagine how they greet you. Feel the love and warmth that emanates from within.

How do you spend your day now? Do you get in your perfect car to drive to your dream job? Do you take a run in your beautiful neighbourhood? Do you spend the morning sculpting your perfect garden? Whatever it is, imagine it all. Imagine the feel of the car seats; the smell of the trees in your neighbourhood; the strength in your running legs; the feel of the soil under your fingers. Imagine the end of the day, with your family sitting around the dinner table, ready to celebrate and honor you with their love and laughter. You share the pride of finally living the dream, which has now become your reality.

It's only from dreams like this that the limitless potential within you will be able to shine. Without it, it will always remain dormant and you will never see your ultimate expression. Most of us have lost our childlike wonder somewhere along the way. We have allowed our life circumstances and our destructive belief patterns to shut the door to dreaming.

It doesn't matter what your dream is. What matters is taking ownership of it. Once you truly own it and believe that you deserve this, the path then becomes illuminated.

You're the only one that has the key to unleash your dreams and place them into action. Now is the time to play the lead role in your life and allow yourself to live out your dreams. Now is the time to stop comparing yourself to others. Now is the time to spend your energy planning your dreams.

Today is a new day, a completely blank page. It's a day for you to create the life of your dreams. Pick up a pen, take a few deep breaths, sit quietly and allow yourself to truly feel the life you want. What have you always dreamed of achieving, but haven't been able to? What would you do if excuses didn't exist? Write it out in the space below. Don't hold back – no one else has to see this. This is for you and you alone.

_____

_____

_____

_____

_____

This dream life is going to be your motivation throughout the next 13 weeks. It's going to be what ignites your fire and lets you stand your ground to become the powerful leader within your life. This is REAL Motivation - motivation that comes from you and no one else.

You deserve this life, but more importantly, you are the only one that is able to fulfill this life. The key that is waiting to unlock the hidden life that is truly you.

In this section you will examine your life right now to uncover the path to your dream life. You will discover how you can become fearless and the strength that's already within you to achieve your dreams. You will fill out a REAL Motivation card, which will form the foundation of your fearless journey over the next 13 weeks. Use it to ignite your fire to pursue the dreams that you deserve!

Getting REAL

Getting REAL with your life is a process of examining and reflecting on your actions, thoughts and behaviors. This will help you become aware and in control of your life. You are the lead character and you call the shots. With this exercise, you get to write your own life story.

Reality

Events

Attitude

Let it go

R = Reality

To begin this process, you must examine a few things within your life. Don't rush it. You have to be fully committed to yourself to really see and, yes, sometimes it takes looking at the skeletons in the closet so you can overcome them. Keep in mind that this is the first step to real positive change - get excited!

You will have to allow 10 minutes or more for this first exercise, so please ensure you have undisturbed time. Find a space that you are comfortable in. Close your eyes and take 10 deep breaths, filling your lungs with air. Exhale through your nose. With each exhalation, relax your body. If you are not relaxed after 10 breaths, continue for another seven.

As with the exercise at the beginning of this chapter, observe yourself with your mind's eye as if you were watching a movie. This time, however, you're going to be looking at your present life, the way it is right now. Just sit back and watch. Don't judge, don't get angry; just allow what is being played out to happen.

As you watch yourself on this screen, what character traits are you showing? Reflect on why you are not living your dreams. Below are some of the common character traits you might see, and ways you can overcome them.

The Victim: Stand up for yourself; don't allow others to use their power on you.

The Child: Resist acting out in ways that are childlike. Practice being selfless.

The Self-Sabotager: Start believing in yourself and change your negative self-talk.

The Workaholic: Why do you work so hard? Take a realistic look at your career obligations and balance your life.

The Servant: You become empowered when you serve your own needs and trust yourself opposed to others.

The Addict: Your own power is the most important thing in your life. Use your own power to examine and begin overcoming your addictions.

The Excuser: It's normal to be afraid of new situations, but be brave! Think of how proud you'll be of yourself when you step out of your comfort zone.

The Rescuer: You care deeply about your family and friends' happiness. Let them live their own lives - mistakes are the best way to learn.

The Disciplinarian: Life experience is what makes us who we are. Past mistakes or failures are just that - in the past. Learn from them instead of beating yourself up over them.

The Procrastinator: Starting something new can be overwhelming, but it doesn't have to be! Taking even a small step towards achieving what you want to accomplish will bring you an immense sense of relief and you'll see how easy it is!

The Disguiser: Being honest with yourself is difficult, but self-awareness is the key to change. Honestly examine the reasons behind your actions and don't be afraid!

E = Events

Once you have watched yourself in your movie, you can find your events - things you are doing. Look for events that have happened in the past that led you to this life you are now living. What patterns have you created? What type of masks or disguises are you wearing? Did you have a strict upbringing? Did you feel lonely growing up? Did you have an abusive relationship? These are all events that can create the patterns that you are now living.

A = Attitude

What attitude are you carrying around? What belief system? What are you telling yourself? Some beliefs I've heard often are: "My family's happiness comes before my own," "Spending money on myself is wasteful," "I'm not strong enough to ask for that promotion" "Once I've taken care of a few other things, then I'll finally travel" and "Maybe I don't deserve my dream." Do any of these phrases sound familiar? These are all attitudes that do not need to hold you back!

L = Let it Go

I know how hard it is to face certain aspects about yourself that only you know about. We are too insecure to share our deepest thoughts and feelings with anyone for fear of being judged, and having labels placed on us. Let it go! It's time to move forward!

26

This is the fun part. Now that you have taken an honest look at your life at this moment, you can begin to create your new reality and take steps toward your dreams.

Get REAL Again

This time, instead of watching the past, you watch the future. What is it that you want? Where is it that you want to go? Remember, this is the part in the movie where it really gets exciting, where you begin to see the plot change. You know, where in all action movies the story begins to turn around? Yes that part. The hero's luck begins to change and the hero begins to take control.

Now it's your turn. You are not only the lead character in this movie, but also the writer. You have the choice at this moment to change any aspect of your life. How are you going to have this played out? Again, take your time and go through the same process as before. Ensure that you have some time alone where you will not be disturbed. Take your deep breaths as before, and now recreate or write a new story.

Remember to take your time with this. This is your life and we need to be conscious enough to create our new reality. All movie characters have to overcome adversities in order to change their direction in life. It's about knowing and having faith within you, to create a new reality.

See yourself on the screen. With your outcome in mind, where does this movie lead you? What events are taking place to help with your transformation? Is there something that jumps out at you? How does it end?

With this exercise, you have the opportunity to change any component of your life. Remember, we all need time to evolve. Our habits didn't form overnight; they evolved over time and that is the same with our lives. Each step we take enables our lives to change. Now that you have watched the movie again, become REAL all over again:

R = Reality

Examine your chosen area in a scenario where everything is the way you want it to be. You may finally be in school, maybe have that promotion, or your able to run the marathon you've been dreaming about. How does the story end?

E = Events

What is happening in this new scenario? What new, helpful patterns have you created? What action steps do you need in order to make this your reality?

A = Attitude

What attitude do you need to maintain your new situation? What belief system has shifted? Choose three power words to help you attain that ideal attitude and remind you of your goal. Examples: confidence, adventurous, attentive, committed, courage, determined, enthusiasm, genuine, inquisitive, inspirational, powerful, honest, integrity, and many more.

L = Let it In

Let this in – own it! You can have this! You are ready mentally and spiritually to make a change, not just physically. You have forgiven yourself or others and are ready to make a fresh start with no past issues to hold you back.

Your REAL Motivation Card (Pg. 30)

Now that you have reflected on your past and thought about what you want in the future, fill out the REAL Motivation card. By getting REAL, you are focusing your energy to become motivated in the area of your life that you wish to transform.

Reality: Write what it is that you want.
Event: What action steps do you need to do in order to attain this?
Attitude: Choose three power words that will help you shift your belief system.
Let it in: Own it and believe in it.

You need to find a picture or image that represents the area of your life that you have chosen to change. You can find this picture in a magazine or it might be a picture from your past. It could even be multiple ones - a collage, if you will. Now that you have a picture of your vision, write down three action steps that you will need in order to attain this. If there are more than three, write the first three and then complete another card when you have completed the first three steps.

Last but not least, write your three power words on your card. Say them as many times throughout the day that is needed. Take this card with you. Keep it in your wallet, at work, or even make a few, and place them around your house; whatever works to help you stay motivated.

By getting REAL you have uncovered your REAL Motivation. Look at both your answers on getting REAL and you will see that they are opposite. They are complete mirror images of each other. REAL Motivation *is your vision in motion*.

Take this card with you wherever you go and refer to it often. Review it before or after your workouts. Use it to remind yourself that you are fueling your inner fire, the inner fire that will help you succeed in achieving your dreams. Refer to it when you want to give up as a reminder to yourself what you need to do to own your dream. You'll find that the last set, the last run up the hill or the last 15 minutes of your workout might not be as hard as you think! Align yourself with your REAL Motivation and you will become your own inspiration.

I suggest over the next 13 weeks you decide on three areas in your life you would like to transform, using this REAL Motivation technique. By using this you will be able to tap into your spirit and find the courage and strength to change your beliefs and habits to free yourself from the past. Every four weeks, complete a new REAL Motivation card with your intent for the following month. Be sure to acknowledge your accomplishments each week. Some examples of three areas for transforming are: your body; saving money; getting our of debt; or maybe even making a step into a new career.

There are more ideas in Chapter 2- Your Life Blueprint.

Create a REAL Motivation Board

Take what you've learned in your REAL Motivation exercise and create a special place to keep yourself inspired. Use a bulletin board or even a sheet of paper that you can refer to every day. Find photos, quotes and other images that relate to the reality you envision for yourself. Each day, look at your REAL Motivation board and let the images inspire you to make your dreams a reality. You are always evolving and developing. Keep working on your motivation.

REAL Motivation

REALITY	EVENTS	ATTITUDE	LET IT GO/IN

THE PAST

THE FUTURE

Getting REAL

Add your picture here.

ACTIONS:

_____

_____

_____

POWER WORDS:

_____

_____

_____

In my own life, I used the REAL Motivation principle to transform my body, my career and my relationship with myself. I was able to see the path my life had taken based on my upbringing and my relationship with my family. Through REAL Motivation, I was able to identify why I suffered from addiction and how I gave up on my power. I was able to finally see that I deserved happiness, good health and success, and I was able to chart the course to achieve these dreams.

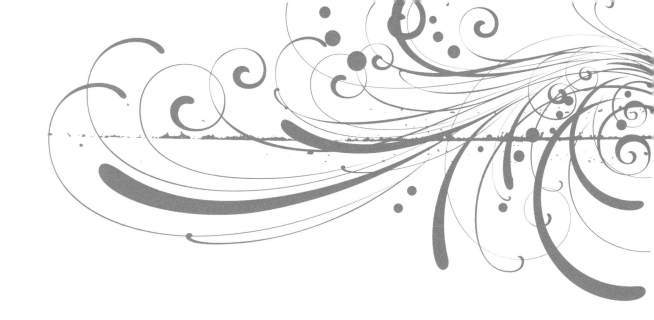

Chapter Three
YOUR LIFE BLUEPRINT

"Our deeds determine us, as much as we
determine our deeds."

George Eliot

YOUR LIFE BLUEPRINT

So far, your life may have been influenced by what your family has set for you. That's okay - our families, whether "good" or "bad," have given each of us lessons we can use. But what really matters, more than our past or how we were raised, is what we do tomorrow. We have a chance to leave a blueprint that will make us proud, one also to be proud to leave for our children.

The following are different components of life that must be examined to achieve balance. If one of these components is off, you may feel it in other areas of your life. Review each one and decide for yourself what standards you'd like to live by. Don't rush this process; allow the thoughts to come to you in their own time. Allow yourself to truly examine what it is that you would like to create for your future.

This exercise is related to, but different from REAL Motivation. REAL Motivation concerns your own personal goals and dreams. Your Life Blueprint is all about the standards and examples you would like to set for yourself and for your loved ones. It's a great exercise for you to do with your spouse or partner as well, whether you have children or not. Like REAL Motivation, reflect on your Life Blueprint every day. Create a time for yourself, to examine this and what you have done that day to further the Life Blueprint you want.

Your Life Blueprint

Prosperity: What belief system would you like to share with your children? What belief system do you need to change? Do you take responsibility for your debt, including loans from family members? Do you allow money to have power over you? Do you allow money to make the decisions in your life? Are you never able to have enough? What does wealth mean to you?

Career: Are you doing something you love? Are you using your natural born talent? How do you balance work and your life? Are you applying yourself as best you can? Are you taking courses to increase your skills? What do you really want to do?

Health: Are you taking care of yourself in mind, body and spirit? Are you addicted? Do you have a consistent workout regimen? Do you get regular health checkups? How is your posture? Are your meals healthy? Are you feeding your family nutritionally dense food? Do you treat yourself?

Wealth & Success: Do you believe you can be successful? What determines success for you? Is it money? Career? Do you take chances?

Relationships & Family: Do you show love and affection with touch and gestures? Do you encourage your family and friends' success? Do you share your thoughts and feelings with your family? Do you show respect for others opinions? Who are your friends? Are they a good influence on you? Are you inspired by their actions?

Spirituality: What are your beliefs? Do you respect other belief systems? Do you have gratitude for the world we live in? Do you practice meditation? Are you holding onto past pain and hurts? Do you have forgiveness?

Environment: What does your house look like? Are you organized? Do you respect your car, your house, and your wardrobe? Is everyone sharing the responsibility in your home or are you doing everything or nothing?

Soul Practice: Does your family have fun? Do you take trips? Do you take time for family nights? Are these things important to you? Do you have great memories of special occasions or trips? Do you keep traditions or maybe create new ones?

Whether we realize it or not, we are creating this blueprint for our children. I believe in order to change, we must be willing to own our own power and create what it is that we want to leave for the next generation. I believe that if enough of us take responsibility for our Life Blueprint, we can consciously create what will become our children's blueprint.

Create Your Own Life Blueprint

Create your own Life Blueprint and set your standards for the following areas:

Prosperity: _____

_____

_____

_____

Career: _____

_____

_____

_____

Health: _____

_____

_____

_____

Wealth & Success: _____

_____

_____

_____

Relationships & Family: _____

_____

_____

_____

Spirituality: _____

_____

_____

_____

Environment: _____

_____

_____

_____

Soul Practice: _____

_____

_____

_____

Create a Life Blueprint Board

Take what you've written above and use it to inspire yourself every day! Take a large piece of paper or a bulletin board and write out what standards and examples you've decided on for each area of your Life Blueprint. Over the next 13 weeks, add to it whenever something catches your eye that relates to your Life Blueprint. It could be a picture of a neatly organized kitchen from a magazine, a photo of your family or a receipt from a charitable donation you've made - anything that represents your ideal Life Blueprint.

On my own Life Blueprint board is a picture of my daughter and myself. Within my own Life Blueprint, this represents the power of determination for me to change the path that I once lived. Every time I look at this picture, I'm reminded that it's up to me to use the courage found within myself to lead by example.

Get creative and have fun with it! Taking an active role in planning your life will put your dreams into action!

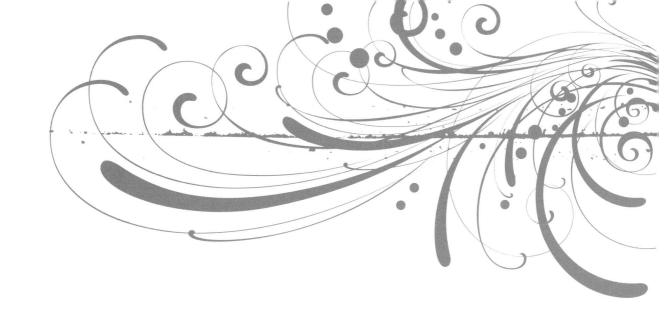

Chapter Four
AFFIRMATIONS

"Quiet minds cannot be perplexed or frightened, but
go on in fortune or misfortune at their own private
pace, like a clock during a thunderstorm."

Robert Louis Stevenson

AFFIRMATIONS

Releasing the Emotional Energy Within

Affirmations are words or phases that help us put our energy into becoming present. They help us to move on with our life, they help us release the past and keep us on track to get what we truly want. Use them to accomplish what you wrote out in your Life Blueprint.

During my initial transformation, I wrote an affirmation on each different area in my life in order to move forward. What I suggest here is that you review the areas listed below and either choose from the list or create your own. You can write your affirmations in the journal section and read them as often as you would like. It's an empowering tool to repeat them in the mirror as well.

Take a deep breath before you read the following affirmations and write down the ones that touch something inside you. You will know by how they make you feel – don't overanalyze. This is your life to create and this is an amazing tool that will help you succeed.

Past:

1. I now release the events of my past. I am at peace.

2. I now face and accept my past with courage and strength.

3. I now forgive myself and others for past actions and mistakes. I am now free.

Present:

1. I love and appreciate myself. I live for this present moment.

2. I am now owning my true self and my abilities.

3. It is safe to be my true self.

Future:

1. I own the power to create endless possibilities for myself.

2. My future is filled with hope, promise and endless prosperity.

3. I allow myself to grow and age with dignity and strength.

Spirituality:

1. I trust and listen to the guidance of my own truth.

2. I allow the beauty of life to fill me.

3. I am on an endless journey. I have the power to create anything!

Health:

1. My body is transforming with each passing day.

2. My posture is tall, my mind is at peace and my spirit is filled with happiness.

3. I nourish my body with life giving foods to provide me with stamina to achieve my dreams.

Relationships and Family:

1. I forgive and accept the relationships of my past. I am at peace.

2. I allow others to make their own path. I see only love.

3. I now give genuine affection and appreciation to my loved ones.

Career:

1. I now have the courage and faith to follow my dreams. All is taken care of.

2. I am fearless in my decisions to embrace my true path.

3. My career fulfills me.

Wealth and Success:

1. I own the power to create wealth and success in my life.

2. I am successful.

3. I am gracefully receiving the wealth and success I truly deserve in my life.

Prosperity:

1. Prosperity comes into my life easily and freely.

2. I now receive graciously the abundance I have created for myself and my future.

3. I now release the emotional attachment of fear and allow true abundance to fill my life.

Environment:

  1. My home is a sacred place, I feel safe and at peace.

  2. I fully appreciate all that is around me.

  3 My home is filled with peace, love and joy!

Soul Practice:

  1. I nurture the traditions of the past and create enduring ones for the future.

  2. My family is surrounded with love and laughter.

  3. Each day is a journey in love.

Create Your Own Affirmations

Write out some of your own affirmations here in the space below. Print them out and keep them with you. Post them in areas where you will see them often, like your car, bedroom, closet or wallet.

Past: _____

_____

_____

_____

_____

Present: _____

_____

_____

_____

_____

Future: _____

_____

_____

_____

_____

Relationships & Family: _____
_____
_____
_____
_____

Career: _____
_____
_____
_____
_____

Wealth & Success: _____
_____
_____
_____
_____

Prosperity: _____
_____
_____
_____
_____

Environment: _____
_____
_____
_____
_____

Soul Practice: _____
_____
_____
_____
_____

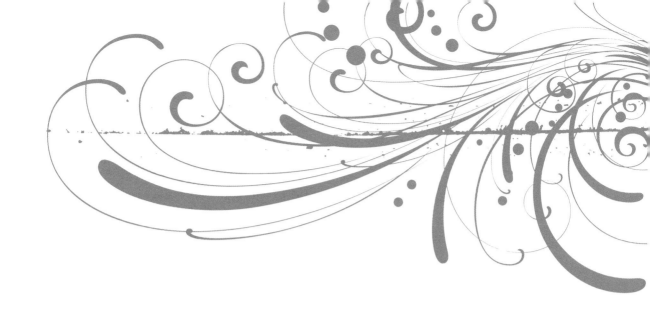

Chapter Five
ORGANIZE YOUR HOME & MIND

"Good order is the foundation of all things."

Edmund Burke

ORGANIZE YOUR HOME & MIND

Now that you have decided on your chosen Life Blueprint, you can clear away your old thought patterns by cleaning out your physical environment. Why is this important? Clearing out your living environment signifies that you are ready to let go of the past, to welcome in new energy of the future.

Many of us neglect our living environments under times of stress or high activity. We become pack rats not releasing old thought patterns, changing our actions or cleaning out our closets. Trust me, if you were to ask my mother, I was a mess growing up - my eating environment, how I took care of my clothes, my messy car. It made sense, considering my life. I know firsthand how good it feels to clear and clean out our physical environment. The environment we live in is just as crucial to the development of our spirit. Be surrounded by love and not toxic environments. Create your safe haven and take responsibility for organizing all areas of your life in a way that brings you peace. The more you're willing to face in the physical world, such as cleaning out your closets, the easier it'll be to do the same with your emotional and mental closets.

Try this activity: Take a tour of your home mentally. Envision your house, closets, garage and basement. How does that make you feel? Are you pleased with what you see? Does your home accurately represent you? Why do you keep things - is it out of obligation or sentimentality? Get rid of anything that does not make you feel good or does not benefit your life.

Throughout the next 13 weeks I suggest you make a goal each week to purge one room or closet in your living environment. The first place to start - and of course it goes hand in hand with this program - is your fridge and pantry. Once you've done that, then I suggest the next place is your own personal closet.

By the end of your program, you will have managed to not only transform your physical body, but you will have also managed to reorganize your home. In order to make room for new habits and create the space for you to succeed with your program, you have to clear out the energy of the old.

Here are some tips to organize your home:

- A good way to start is to break up your environment into the levels that you have: basement, main floor, and upstairs.

- I like to start with the basement or garage, as it seems that's where we have a tendency to put things and forget about them. I know it may seem like a daunting task, however I promise once you go through and purge, you will have a newfound inner energy that will give you the momentum.

- From there, break it down even more into specific rooms on each level.

- Then, make a list of what you need to do with each room.

- Clean out everything. Don't allow one corner or cushion to go unturned, put all of your effort into it.

- Take one step at a time. Be conscious and decide whether what you have is worth keeping. If it feels good then keep it. If not, discard, donate or recycle.

- Do it over time.

- Clean and dust all furniture.

- Clean and wipe your baseboards.

- Make it a family project.

- When cleaning out the closets, remember if you have not worn it chances are you won't, so get rid of it. Allow space for your new wardrobe to enter!

- In the bathrooms, get rid of any product you haven't used. Chances are you don't remember you had it!

Now that you have a schedule when each room is to be done, it's easy to keep on track to do one room a week. You can also get help by enlisting your children and your spouse or partner to help you with it.

When you are finished reorganizing your home you'll feel a renewed energy and ownership over your safe haven. Use this new energy towards reaching your goals in other areas of your life!

Chart and schedule

Living Space:	Responsibility:	When:
Kitchen (More tips for organizing your kitchen can be found in Chapter 8) - Cupboards - Pantry - Stove/Oven - Fridge - Containers - Other		
Dining Room		
Living Room		
Family Room		
Office		
Bathroom (1)		
Bathroom (2)		

Living Space:	Responsibility:	When:
Bedroom (1)		
Bedroom (2)		
Bedroom (3)		
Closet (1)		
Closet (2)		
Closet (3)		
Gym		
Storage Room		
Finances / Paper Work		
Garage		
Vehicle		
Shed / Outside Storage		
Other		
Other		
Other		

liv

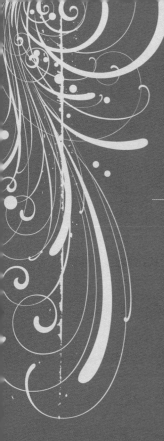

Be Confidence, where there is Confidence there is Enthusiasm and where there is Enthusiasm there is FREEDOM

Body & Nutrition

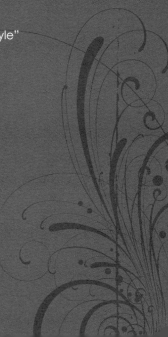

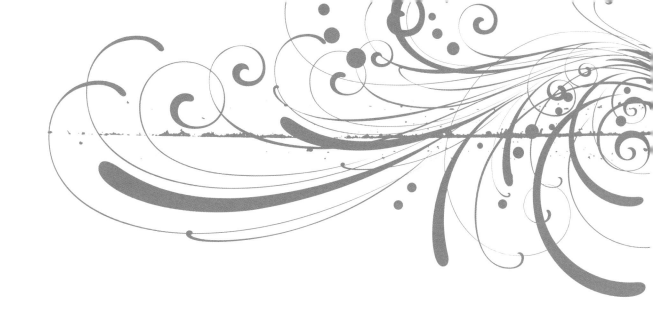

Chapter Six
THE "NUTRITIONAL LIFESTYLE"

"Don't dig your grave with your own knife and fork."

English Proverb

THE "NUTRITIONAL LIFESTYLE"

I have struggled with weight loss, and I'm sure many of you have too. Where do we find the truth with all the different views on what is good for us and what isn't? Where do we even start? It seems all so confusing. I recently heard that by the year 2020, something like 55% of the population will be overweight or obese. Billions of dollars are spent to help these people lose weight. What we need to do is to take ownership of our own nutrition.

Most programs and diets may have started with good intentions, but billion-dollar companies who are all under pressure to outshine their competition own most of them. This results in a wave of quick-fix products that just end up confusing us. What does your intuition tell you? I bet you feel happier thinking about a plate of seasoned chicken, wild rice and colourful vegetables than you do about a handful of pills. Trust this intuition! Create your own to make nutrition a whole-life habit and not a band-aid solution. This way, you will approach eating as a way to fuel your body in the way it needs and you will feel revitalized and strong.

Lead by Example

During my weight loss journey, I knew I needed to take control of my life completely, and this included discovering and owning my Nutritional Lifestyle. I was tired from all of my previous failed attempts with my diets, calorie-counting programs, the pills and the powders. I wanted to break free from the emotional relationship I had with food and I was not going to allow my daughter to repeat my struggles and roadblocks with food and weight loss.

We all deserve and need to be healthy. However, there comes a time when we need to make lifestyle changes that are not only for ourselves, but for our children - a legacy wherein we will teach our children the right eating habits to continue throughout their entire lives. We need to stand up and take the lead. We need to be the role models in our children's lives. We need to take responsibility for our own Nutritional Lifestyle.

I will never forget one afternoon when my husband and daughter were running errands. It was around lunchtime when they returned. My daughter came rushing into the house saying, "Mommy Mommy, guess what? Daddy had a hamburger!"

I thought for sure that he would have bought her a children's meal. When I asked my daughter what she had, she replied, "Nothing Mommy. I wanted to come home and have something healthy, because fast food is not healthy!"

I was so proud of her, a four-year-old turning down fast food.

When it comes to our bodies, I feel that each and every one of us should take the responsibility for it. A Nutritional Lifestyle is "Leading by Example".

Creating Your Nutritional Lifestyle

A Nutritional Lifestyle is an overall balance of your eating habits, your emotional connection to them, and a basic understanding of the foods you eat to ensure you are properly energizing your body. Here are some questions I want you to think about before you create Your Nutritional Lifestyle.

When was the last time you and your family sat at the table and thoroughly enjoyed your meal, with no distractions and no rushing?
When was the last time you planned your meal ahead of time?
When was the last time you made your lunch the night before?
When was the last time you tried a new recipe or bought a new vegetable?
When was the last time you listened to your body when you were full?
When was the last time you prepared a meal with nothing but fresh, real ingredients?

Obstacles to Overcome

Aside from the barrage of quick-fix weight loss products, there is another nutritional obstacle that's a bit tougher to handle: "addictions". Addictions to food, alcohol, smoking, drugs, sex or gambling - they're all the same. In my own life, I experienced a couple of these addictions.

It started with smoking at the age of 15. I was a closet smoker for over eight years. I also dealt with my drug addiction from the ages of 18 to 21. Throughout my life I also faced the addiction to food.

The addiction to food became stronger over the years. At first it was somewhat normal eating. Then it progressed into intense overeating sessions, then into exercise bulimia, and then into full-out bulimia. Eventually I was at a point where I was so controlled by "it" that I would have four binge and purge sessions a day.

As intense as it was, I was not going to go back to see a therapist. This addiction was here to teach me something. I needed to do my own research and understand why this intense desire to eat kept coming over me.

During my research, I read that most people who have an eating disorder come from a family where alcoholism or sexual trauma has taken place. For me, that made sense. I grew up with domestic abuse, alcoholism as well as sexual trauma.

It took a few months, but I was finally able to understand and acknowledge the energy I felt when the addiction came over me. I learned how I could feel the addiction without giving in to it, because if I had even one thing in my mouth when I was in that state I would not be able to stop.

I'm not suggesting that addiction treatment or therapy should be ignored. Please, if you think you're suffering from an addiction, talk to your doctor. But for me personally, I was able to take my power back from my addiction to food and bring it back to myself. This awareness of the signs and cravings gave me the power I needed to work through each one.

Don't get me wrong - it wasn't an easy journey. Sometimes I gave in to my intense cravings. I couldn't stop thinking about food. My mind wanted more and more. I almost didn't care what I was eating and why - I just wanted to eat. Then, of course, came the guilt and hateful thoughts.

I was very overwhelmed by the energy I felt. This negative energy was very intense and, at times, seemed like my entire identity. After a lot of struggle and self-reflection, I realized I was more than my addiction to food. I discovered what emotions triggered my eating and purging episodes and what I needed to do to overcome them.

Here are a few signs from my past that the addiction was around:

- I became agitated.
- Intense feelings of energy surrounded by food.
- All I could think about was eating.
- I wanted more before I was even done.
- The knowledge that I was about to eat made me elated.
- I was not craving one particular food or flavor, but several.

Here are a few things that might trigger the episodes:

- Negative self-talk.
- Questioning your actions or decisions.
- The feeling that you have to fish for compliments.
- A messy living environment.
- Judgmental thoughts of yourself or others.
- Low self-esteem.
- Lack of commitment to your dreams.
- Procrastination over your desired plans.
- Lack of organization.
- Over thinking.
- Always waiting for the next thing to happen.
- Living either in the past or the future.
- Not taking responsibility for your actions.
- Not owning your own power, or words.
- Rushing through things to get them done.
- Being a perfectionist.
- Passively allowing your life to happen - one day becomes the same as the next.
- Giving people with higher levels of education or experience more authority over you.
- Resisting or becoming irritated by tasks we need to perform.

What I've experienced is the more you give into your own addiction, the more power you give to "it." So what do we do? We get on with our lives. We take back our own power. The more power we have in the present to create our lives, the less of a chance our addictions have to do it for us.

Here are techniques you can add to your eating regimen to help you:

- Place food in your mouth only at meal and snack times.
- Eat only while sitting down.
- Prepare your food with love and attention to all of the wonderful nutrition that your body will receive from it.
- Set the table to reflect respect for this relationship.
- Become grounded or be present before you eat.
- Give thanks for the wondrous foods that you are about to eat.
- Think about the lovely colours of your food and what steps it took to get to your plate.
- Bring your attention to the taste and texture of the food you are eating.
- Eat slowly and mindfully.

Take ownership of your Nutritional Lifestyle and allow it to direct your life. Creating healthy habits and attitudes towards food will mirror the respect you will feel towards your own body. This respect and ownership will put you in the driver's seat to your best life.

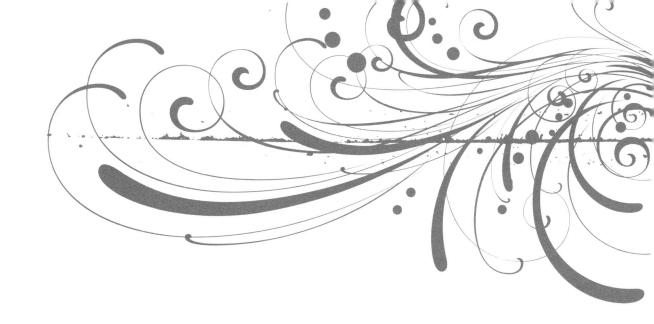

Chapter Seven
ABOUT NUTRITION

"To eat is a necessity, but to eat intelligently is an art."

La Rochefoucauld

ABOUT NUTRITION

In this chapter, we'll take a look at what food really does for you. Knowing the basics about nutrition and understanding the more technical terms will help you take ownership of your "Nutritional Lifestyle".

First, let's take a look at some myths and misconceptions surrounding nutrition.

Myths and Misconceptions about Nutrition

Working with as many women and men as I have, I've heard some interesting things about food over the years. These myths and misconceptions when followed, cause harm and damage to the human body, and become roadblocks on the path to a healthy mind and spirit as well.

Myth: *I need to lose 10 pounds, maybe I should do a cleanse?*
Truth: Cleanses are great but not for losing weight. In order to prevent the yo-yo of weight gain/loss, focus on eating only nutritious food, exercising regularly and getting enough rest. It will save you pain and frustration.

Myth: *I'll just fill up on raw veggies.*
Truth: Well, for starters we need to eat to sustain life and we should be eating to nourish our bodies and our souls. Filling up on veggies only is restricting the other essential components of nutrition that our bodies need and it also inhibits the joy that a varied, healthy "Nutritional Lifestyle" can bring you.

Myth: *Olive oil is healthy, does it matter how much I use?*
Truth: Olive oil is good, but just because something is good for us does not mean we can eat as much as we want. Enjoy your olive oil, but enjoy it in moderation.

Myth: *I eat breakfast, lunch and dinner. I was taught that three square meals a day is all I need.*
Truth: Your body is similar to a car, in the sense that it requires frequent stops for fuel to keep running optimally. Eating five to six small meals every two to three hours, with a serving of carbs, paired with either a protein, a fat or both, is actually

the best way to keep your energy up and your metabolism working for you. For example, pair an apple with a handful of nuts or a serving of cottage cheese paired with fresh fruit. This will keep your energy up and blood sugar levels balanced.

Myth: *I don't have time for breakfast. I'll just grab a latte.*
Truth: Skipping breakfast is not the best idea for anyone. You've been sleeping all night and your body needs fuel to get you through the day. By eating breakfast within 60 minutes of waking you prime your metabolism for the day. Think of it this way: It's -20 degrees in the middle of winter, would you just turn on the engine of your car and drive? I don't think so. You need to let your car warm up. This is the same thing with your metabolism. Breakfast turns on your metabolic "engine".

Myth: *I need coffee to get through my day.*
Truth: When we feel tired, it's often because we are lacking proper hydration or energy. Grab a friend, two bottles of water, and head outside for an H2O break. Walk around the block, walk to your favourite park or even just walk the stairs. You will get the same effect as that afternoon coffee - even better, actually.

Myth: *I can't lose weight. I lost 20 pounds but I just gained it all back.*
Truth: I have met so many women and men who have tried all of these crash diets. They may help you lose weight fast, but they are so dangerous. Calorie-reduced diets slow down your metabolism temporarily. When you return to eating normally, your metabolism has adjusted to eating fewer calories, meaning you gain weight again. Crash diets also make you go on a damaging cycle of unhappiness and discouragement. Small reductions of about 500 calories per day is recommended. Keep in mind that weight loss of more than one to two pounds per week is not healthy and may stress your body in dangerous ways. Create a "Nutritional Lifestyle" and break the chain.

ABOUT MACRONUTRIENTS & MICRONUTRIENTS

They may sound fancy, but you deal with macronutrients and micronutrients every day of your life. What are they? Macronutrients are carbohydrates, proteins and fat. Micronutrients are vitamins, minerals and water.

MACRONUTRIENTS

CARBOHYDRATES

Carbohydrates are critical to the health of both your body and your mind. Did you know that they are used as fuel by every part of your body and are the only source of energy for your brain?

Carbs come in two forms: complex and simple. Complex carbohydrates are high in fiber, help you feel full longer and keep your energy stable. Vegetables, unrefined grains (such as oats and brown rice) and whole grain products are complex carbohydrates.

On the other hand, simple carbohydrates digest quickly and absorb into the body rapidly. Fruits and vegetables are a source of simple carbohydrates providing natural sugar and important vitamins and minerals. Other less nutritious simple sugars include refined grains, high fructose corn syrup, pop and processed/packaged foods. Generally speaking, these foods provide very little nutrition other than empty calories.

liv

PROTEIN

Protein is vital in maintaining, repairing and rebuilding all tissues and muscles. It transports fluids and oxygen to every part of your body. Proteins create hormones and enzymes for your immune system.

FATS

Fat is an important source of energy for the body. They contribute to healthy skin and the production of hormones. They also transport fat-soluble vitamins throughout your body. Fats come in three types: saturated, unsaturated and trans fats. Saturated fats are solid at room temperature and are primarily found in animal products such as cheese and butter. They may increase cholesterol levels. Unsaturated fats are liquid at room temperature. They are derived from plant sources and are the healthier fat to consume. Trans fats should be avoided as they are unnatural, synthetic fat. These include hydrogenated and partially hydrogenated oils.

MICRONUTRIENTS

VITAMINS

Have you ever wondered what's in that multivitamin you take and what everything does for you? Let's take a look at the vitamins we need.

Our bodies use 13 different vitamins. Vitamins are taken from food to regulate activities in different areas of your body. Water-soluble vitamins, such as B complex and C, come out in your urine regularly and must be replaced often by the food you eat. Fat soluble vitamins, such as A, D, E and K are stored in your organs and body fat.

Glycemic Index Foods

You may have heard the phrase "glycemic index," or GI. This refers to the affect that certain carbohydrates have on our blood glucose levels. High GI foods release glucose quickly and raise your blood sugar quickly as well. Low GI foods release glucose steadily over hours so you feel full longer. What it comes down to is the proper food to sustain you all day long. Why would you want to go up with a rush of sugar and then down? I would rather just be in balance, how about you?

Examples of high GI foods include simple carbs like white bread, donuts and cornflakes. Examples of low GI foods include complex carbs, such as whole grain bread, yogurt and chickpeas. As I mentioned earlier in this chapter, simple carbs are digested quicker, are often refined and less nutritious. Complex carbs are fiber-rich, keep you feeling full longer and help your blood glucose levels stay stable.

Basal Metabolic Rate

Your basal metabolic rate (BMR) is the number of calories your body requires to function on a basic level, without you performing any activity. These are the calories your body uses to breathe, sleep, pump blood and other vital actions you often aren't even conscious of.

Part of owning your Nutritional Lifestyle is taking the role of ownership with your life. I believe that each one of us should know our BMR to help us understand what our bodies require to sustain life.

Calculate Your BMR

Here is a formula you can use to calculate your basal metabolic rate. This number is just an estimate. A number of other factors, such as genetics and age, can affect your BMR, but it will give you a better idea of what you really need to fuel your body.

Males = 66 + (13.7 x weight in kg) + (5 x height in cm) - (6.8 x age)

Females = 655 + (9.6 x weight in kg) + (1.8 x height in cm) - (4.7 x age)

So, for a woman weighing 68 kg, who is 170 cm tall and 34 years of age, her formula would look like this:
655 + (9.6 x 68) + (1.8 x 170) - (4.7 x 34)

Making her BMR 1,454. This is the number of calories she needs to simply exist.

Calculate yours here: _____

Now, that you know you BMR, apply this Harris Benedict Equation for the activity factor and calculate your body's daily caloric requirements:

1. If you are sedentary (little or no exercise): BMR x 1.2
2. If you are lightly active (light exercise/sports 1-3 days per week): BMR x 1.375
3. If you are moderately active (moderate exercise/sports 3-5 days per week): BMR x 1.55
4. If you are very active (hard exercise/sports 6-7 days per week): BMR x 1.725
5. If you are extra active (very hard exercise/sports and physical job or 2x training) BMR x 1.9

My need: _____calories

How to Read Nutritional Information Panels and Labels

Ah, the confusing world of nutritional information. You probably know that you should read nutritional information and package labels, but you might not be sure what to look for. Don't worry — it's easier than you might think.

WATER SOLUBLE VITAMINS

THIAMIN (B1) - Found in liver, pork, wheat germ, whole grains, enriched breads & cereals, legumes and nuts. Assists with nervous system and in carbohydrate metabolism.

RIBOFLAVIN (B2) - Found in milk products, liver, enriched breads and cereals. Promotes good vision and healthy skin; metabolizes protein and energy.

NIACIN (B3) - Found in liver, poultry, fish, peanut butter, legumes and mushrooms. Contributes to healthy skin, nerves and gastrointestinal tract.

PANTOTHENIC ACID (B5) - Found in eggs, liver, wheat bran, peanuts, legumes, meat, spinach and other vitamins. Assists in energy and tissue metabolism.

PYRIDOXINE (B6) - Found in liver, herring, salmon, wheat germ, whole grains, meats, legumes, bananas. Assists in red blood cell production and protein and fat metabolism.

FOLIC ACID (B9) - Found in liver, wheat bran, whole grains, spinach, dark leafy greens, vegetables, legumes and nuts. Assists in red blood cell production, regulates tissue processes, helps metabolize carbs and protein. It's also very important for pregnant women as it helps prevent birth defects.

COBALAMIN (B12) - Found in animal-origin foods. Vegetarian sources are specially prepared fermented yeast, fortified soy products and eggs. It assists metabolism and in the maintenance of red blood cells, nerve tissue and energy.

BIOTIN (H) - Found in organ meats, mushrooms and legumes. Used for the production of fatty acids, metabolism of amino acid, carbs and fat and the maintenance of nerve tissue.

VITAMIN C - Found in citrus, strawberries, cantaloupe, tomatoes, broccoli, potatoes, cabbage and sweet potatoes. Contributes to bone and wound healing; absorbs iron; and increases infection resistance.

FAT SOLUBLE VITAMINS

VITAMIN A - Found in liver, egg yolks, dairy products, yellow vegetables, apricot, cantaloupe. Helps to maintain the health of eyes and skin and contributes to infection resistance.

VITAMIN D - Found in fortified milk and dairy products, cereal, eggs. Helps to absorb calcium and contributes to healthy skin.

VITAMIN E - Found in food with wheat germ and vegetable oils, toasted almonds, roasted sunflower seeds and almond butter. Protects cells, vitamins and fats from destruction.

VITAMIN K - Found in cabbage, cauliflower, leafy greens and vegetables. Promotes blood clotting and bone strength.

MINERALS
Minerals are also simple, but very important. They help with many body functions. They build bones, create hormones, maintain healthy nerves and regulate your cardiovascular system. Examples of minerals include

The nutritional information panel contains the calories and breakdown of macronutrients and micronutrients in a package. It tells you how much of each nutrient is in a package, based on a 2,000 calorie a day diet. Be sure to check out the serving size – you don't want to eat half a package of something, only to find out the nutritional info is only for a third that amount!

The first half of the label is macronutrients and the second half is micronutrients. A good rule of thumb is to go for foods that are high in fiber, at least three grams, and watch for foods that have high sodium, sugar and fat content.

The list of ingredients is presented in order of highest concentration to lowest concentration. Look for whole grains and ingredients that you can pronounce or recognize - it's an easy way to make sure you are nourishing your body with real food. After all, you wouldn't put glycerol monooleate or sorbitan tristearate in your food at home - let alone in your body!

This information will help you get right down to what these things really mean. If something says it's made with real fruit juice, that's great. Until you read the ingredients list and see real juice as the last ingredient on the list. Sure enough, the first ingredient is sugar in the form of glucose. If something sounds too good to be true, then it is. Learning to read nutritional information labels is easy and will help you take control of your Nutritional Lifestyle.

About Calories and Serving Sizes
Another common roadblock to a Nutritional Lifestyle is knowing and following the correct serving sizes. I found that most people are eating too much of something or not enough. Their meal consisted of only carbohydrates, or protein. To make a balanced "Nutritional Lifestyle" meal pair a carbohydrate with either a protein, fat or both.

Here is a perfect example of a dinner with the right serving of each:

- 1 breaded chicken breast (25% lean proteins)
- 3\4 cup wild rice (25% complex carbohydrates)
- 1 cup of broccoli (50% vegetables)

It all depends on your personal taste. For example, my husband's face when I served him this meal above wasn't too pretty. He liked this one much better:

- Barbecue chicken pita pizza **(recipe on page 259)**
- Fresh garden salad

I was sneaky - he thought he was getting a treat, when in reality they are both equivalent in their breakdown of macronutrients and servings!

Here is a breakdown of what your Nutritional Lifestyle should consist of throughout the day.

1. Carbohydrates = 5-6 servings per day
45% - 65% of total daily caloric needs*
- simple carbohydrates, fruits and veggies
- complex carbohydrates, whole grains

2. Protein = 5-6 servings per day
10% - 35% of total daily caloric needs*
- meat and meat alternatives
- low fat dairy and milk products

3. Fats = 5-6 servings per day
20% - 35% of total daily caloric needs*
- healthy unsaturated fats and oils
- nuts and seeds

calcium (maintains healthy bones and teeth), iron (helps to deliver oxygen to tissues and muscles) and sodium (maintains potassium levels in body fluid).

CALCIUM
Found in dairy products (especially in yogurt, milk and cheese) as well as broccoli. It strengthens your bones and teeth, aids in muscle contraction, blood clotting and nerve transmission. It is easy to ensure you have enough calcium in your "Nutritional Lifestyle", try yogurt as a snack, dip or dressing, or add grated cheese to soup.

IRON
Found in hemoglobin, which carries oxygen to your tissues. Meat sources include beef sirloin, lean ground beef, lamb, chicken and tuna. Non-meat sources include dried apricots prunes, baked beans, kidney beans, raisins, cooked spinach and fortified cereals.

WATER
Our bodies are made up of 68% water. This is incredible! Did you know water is essential for our survival? Water aids in digestion, metabolism and in all your body's reactions. It helps lubricate joints and also assists in waste removal and respiration. So drink your water!

Our bodies are all differently sized and, therefore, need different serving sizes than each other. The good news is you don't need fancy equipment to find out your proper serving size - just use your hand!

A serving of carbohydrates is approximately:
The size of your fist. Example: an apple, potato, 1/2 cup wild rice.

A serving of lean protein is approximately:
The size of your palm. Example: a chicken breast, 1/2 - 1 cup of beans, lentils, yogurt or cottage cheese.

A serving of healthy fats is approximately:
A handful: Example: 10-15 almonds, liquid fats (oils or nut butters) 1-2 tbsp. cheese, the size of two fingers.

* as per Canada Food Guide

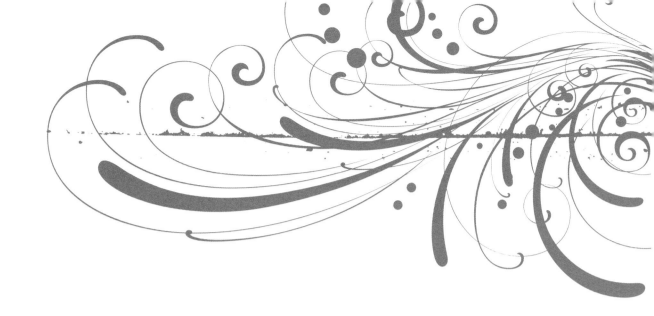

Chapter Eight
DEEPER INTO YOUR "NUTRITIONAL LIFESTYLE"

"The doctor of the future will no longer treat the human frame with drugs, but rather will cure and prevent disease with nutrition."

Thomas Edison

DEEPER INTO YOUR "NUTRITIONAL LIFESTYLE"

Macronutrients and Their Food Groups

In this section, I've tried to make it as easy as possible to understand the right foods to put in your body. Use the list below to help you understand what each food group does for your body.

Each macronutrient fits into one of the major food groups that we are all familiar with. Just in case, they are: Fruits and Veggies; Whole Grains; Milk and Dairy Products; Meat and Poultry; Fats and Oils.

Here is a list of a variety of foods and where each one fits in the macronutrients and the food groups. There are endless possibilities with these healthy food choices. Pick a carb, pair it with a protein, a fat or both to make a meal. It's easy:

Carbohydrates (Complex)
Rice, pasta, grains, breads and cereals

Rice: Brown rice, Wild rice, Brown basmati rice

Pasta: Whole wheat pasta, Couscous

Grains: Kamut, Quinoa, Barley, Spelt

Breads: Sprouted grain , Whole grain, Rye, Pumpernickel

Other: Rice wraps, Whole wheat wraps, Sprouted grain wraps, Whole-wheat pitas, Multigrain rye crackers, Organic seven-grain crackers, Rice cakes, Corn thins

Cereals: Oatmeal, Millet puffs, Rice puffs, Kamut puffs, Whole grain cereals

Starchy Veggies: Baked potato, Sweet potato, Yams, Squash, Pumpkin

Carbohydrates (Simple)
Fruits and Veggies

The amount of veggies you eat is unlimited!

Fruits: Apples, Strawberries, Blueberries, Blackberries, Raspberries, Oranges, Cherries, Peaches, Pears, Plums, Melons, Grapes, Bananas

Other: Apple butter, Applesauce

Veggies: Asparagus, Broccoli, Cabbage, Cauliflower, Cucumber, Dark leafy greens, Mushrooms, Onions, Peppers, Zucchini, Lettuce, Carrots, Green beans, Spinach, Tomato, Snow peas, Brussels sprouts, Artichokes, Celery, Eggplant

Lean Proteins

Fish: Salmon, Tuna, Shrimp, Lobster, Crab, Sole, Trout

Meat & Poultry: Chicken breast, Turkey breast, Lean ground turkey, Lean ground beef, Top sirloin steak

Vegetarian Proteins

Beans and Lentils: Kidney beans, Chickpeas, Black beans, Green/Brown/Red lentils

Other: Edamame beans, Soya burgers, Textured Vegetable Protein, Hemp seeds

Dairy: Cottage cheese (low fat), Eggs, Egg whites or substitutes, Low fat yogurt

Healthy Fats

Nuts and Seeds: Almonds, Cashews, Peanuts, Pumpkin seeds, Sesame seeds, Walnuts

Oils: Flaxseed oil, Olive oil, Safflower oil, Canola oil, Sunflower oil, Coconut oil, Sesame oil, Hempseed oil

Butters: Almond butter, Peanut butter, Cashew butter

Other: Avocados, Low-fat dairy products such as cheese and sour cream

THINGS TO KEEP IN MIND

The safe way to lose weight is one to two pounds per week. 1 lb. = 3500 calories.

Decrease your fat and sugar intake. Use low-fat cooking techniques. Eat low-fat dairy. Choose snacks like fruit and vegetables. Eat small, frequent meals. Drink lots of water. Plan meals in advance. Eat slowly. Avoid commercial weight loss products.

THINK LONG TERM AND CREATE A NUTRITIONAL LIFESTYLE AS OPPOSED TO A QUICK WEIGHT-LOSS DIET.

liv

Soul Meals

An ideal Nutritional Lifestyle is an overall balance of our eating habits. And, yes, this includes treating ourselves. I enjoy chocolate cake, so this is my treat. We need to make sure that we are in balance with what I call soulful eating. Depending on how many meals a day you eat, you're looking at 35-42 meals a week. Why should you deny yourself a little treat for all of these meals? Moderation and balance revitalizes your mind and spirit. I call these healthy treat meals "Soul Meals."

Your Nutritional Lifestyle should be looked at over a span of either a week or even a month. This way you have a better idea of where you are going to use your Soul Meals. Do you meet with friends every Thursday night? Do you have an upcoming dinner party? Maybe you want to use your Soul Meal for your favourite restaurant. Just remember to take at least one to three Soul Meals per week. Remember, serving size counts!

Here are a few tips!

- Eat before you actually feel hungry. This will help your metabolism stay up all day long.

- Eat five to six small meals throughout the day, every two to three hours, with a serving of carbs, protein and fats.

- Working your new eating plan into your daily schedule is possible. Look for healthy choices at restaurants or plan to eat out for your special Soul Meal.

- Who wants to count calories? Just pay attention to your serving sizes. Ensure you are getting the correct serving size of each macronutrient at every meal.

- Don't give up! If you feel overwhelmed, remember this is a lifestyle change and with any kind of change we need to take it one step at a time.

- Have a household calendar on your fridge. On this calendar, place everything that is coming up for that month. You can include your children's schedules, appointments, social events, etc. From there create or use the weekly planner.

- Prepare what you'll cook for the week, considering your plans and events. This will ensure that you're ready and prepared ahead of time to allow the week to go as smoothly as possible.

- Plan for meals and any upcoming events. On Sundays, I prepare for the week ahead to ensure that I have the time and space within me to have dinner with my family.

Cleaning Out Your Fridge

Set yourself up for success. You can't start your Nutritional Lifestyle without having your pantry and fridge conducive to healthy, real food. Getting rid of junk and cleaning out your space is important emotionally, mentally and physically to release the old patterns, and to prepare yourself and your family for this new lifestyle. With all the ingredients you need for the week, you will ensure your transition to a Nutritional Lifestyle will be a success.

To begin with, take everything out of your fridge. By everything I mean everything - drawers, crumbs and all of those old condiments that you've had for years.

Next, separate your fridge into sections (bins from the dollar store are great for this) with the following food groups:

- Meats and poultry. Normally it is just luncheon meat, but this is also the home of any leftovers.
- Fruits.
- Veggies. I separate a small drawer for my onions and herbs.
- Milk and dairy.
- Nuts and seeds. I like to use glass jars.
- Grains. If you like, keep your bread in the fridge.
- Lunches. You can designate a shelf or bin.

Now, begin to sort. Really examine what you have been feeding yourself and your family. Read the labels, read the expiry dates and recycle or reuse what you don't need. Only put back in the fridge what belongs in each bin. This is a great family game to get everyone on board with this lifestyle change.

Your fridge is now set up to help you put your groceries away easier, stay organized and keep on top of your nutrition.

Your freezer is next! Remove everything from it entirely and create spaces that correspond to each of the sections in your fridge. I suggest adding an area for prepared frozen dinners. This is a designated area with in your freezer that already has a few Ticket Meals in place - meals you can use as a freebie in lieu of cooking. Use your Ticket Meals on days where something has come up and you don't have time to cook.

Areas of your freezer:
- Fruits
- Veggies
- Meats
- Grains
- Ticket Meals

Cleaning Out Your Pantry

You can predict what to do now - remove everything from every area of the pantry. Don't just tidy it up. Take it out so you can have a good look at what is in there.

Create sections in your pantry as well. A shelf, bin or even just designated areas will be just fine. Here are the sections for your pantry:

- Breakfast grains and cereals
- Crackers and snacks
- Grains, pastas and rice
- Canned beans, stewed tomatoes, spaghetti sauces, any dinner helpers
- Spices. These are great; you can change the dish by adding some spice.

Label each section and then begin to put your pantry back together. Take a good look at whatever is left and decide what you want to keep or donate.

This is a lot of work, but I promise it will help you with this transition into your new Nutritional Lifestyle. You have begun to take ownership of your new life!

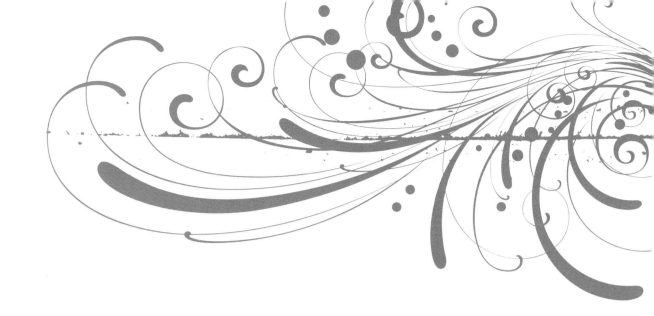

Chapter Nine
HAVING FUN IN THE KITCHEN

"Did you ever stop to taste a carrot? Not just eat it, but
taste it? You can't taste the beauty and energy
of the earth in a Twinkie."

Astrid Alauda

HAVING FUN IN THE KITCHEN

Tips for Grocery Shopping

You now have a fresh start. You have cleared out a space for all the healthy food you need to begin your Nutritional Lifestyle. Now you have to get ready and go shopping.

Most of us use recycled cloth bags and such, but with this program I recommend using bins. At some grocery store chains you can purchase grocery bins, but you can also find bins at any home hardware store that collapse and lie completely flat. They help you stay organized and make it easier to go from the grocery store directly into your fridge.

Just like the fridge and freezer, you are going to have a bin for the following food groups: Fruits, Veggies, Meats and Poultry, Grains, Milk and Dairy, Fats and Oils. Organize yourself with foods you like that are healthy and nourishing. Think about foods in each of the food groups that the whole family enjoys and base your shopping list around that. You can even have your child ask for one item in each food group. This not only encourages them to eat healthy but also makes them feel part of the family.

Here is an example of a grocery store list from my house, made up of favourite foods from my entire family:

Carbohydrates:		
Whole Grain Breads, Pasta, Rice *Bread* *Wraps* *Rice cakes*	Veggies *Cauliflower* *Broccoli* *Spinach* *Radishes*	Fruit *Apples* *Bananas* *Grapes* *Pears*
Lean Proteins:		**Healthy Fats:**
Dairy *Milk* *Yogurt* *Cheese* *Cottage cheese*	Meat | Poultry | Fish | Seafood *Lean turkey breast* *Chicken breasts* *Lean ground beef* *Salmon*	Oils | Nuts | Seeds *Olive Oil* *Walnuts* *Almonds*
Condiments: *Mayonnaise* *Mustard* *Salad dressing*	**Other:** *Bottled Water*	**Household:** *Laundry Detergent* *Paper Towel*

You have your kitchen and grocery store list ready and you are now living your Nutritional Lifestyle. You are now ready to go shopping and fill your bins. To make it extra easy – and fun if you're bringing kids along – write your list on the side of your bins with a dry-erase marker.

Some quick side notes: make sure that you're headed to the grocery store during their slower times. Going shopping in peak times can be stressful and make you feel rushed and irritated. On weekends, try hitting the store as soon as it opens. I also like to make a routine out of it. For me, every Saturday morning is grocery-shopping day. Oh, and please don't go on an empty stomach!

How to Shop at the Grocery Store

No matter how tiny or gigantic your local grocery store is it can be intimidating with the variety of products in each aisle. As you now own your new Nutritional Lifestyle, you are ready to embark on this new adventure with a new set of eyes. Remember you have cleared the energy in your kitchen to only bring home natural food that fits into your life. You have your list and your bins, and the biggest thing to remember is to stay present. Stay focused and don't allow yourself to become distracted with marketing gimmicks, unnecessary aisle wandering or sale items.

With all of the grocery store tours I conducted with my clients I found that most store layouts are the same. Around the perimeter is where you will find most of your items. It might take you a little longer the first time, but you can even make it a little game to beat your time each shopping trip. Just make it fun!

What I like to do is have my daughter help me fill each bin with all of our favourites. If you have more than one child, then each child can take a bin. The fabulous thing about shopping this way is that there is no room in your cart for unhealthy or old-pattern thinking, and you are taking the lead to set an example for your children.

Photocopy the sample shopping list on the following page and use it to stay focused the next time you visit the grocery store.

Carbohydrates:		
Whole Grain Breads, Pasta, Rice, etc.	Veggies	Fruit

Lean Proteins:		Healthy Fats:
Dairy	Meat | Poultry | Fish | Seafood	Oils | Nuts | Seeds

Condiments:	Other:	Household:

Here are a few tips on what to look for in each section:

Produce: Always begin your shopping trip in the produce section. Buy from the back of each shelf - that's where all the freshest fruits and veggies are. Choose a variety of colours to ensure your body receives a wide range of nutrients.

Dairy: Look for low-fat or 1%. Be sure to check expiry dates!

Grains: Your pasta, rice, bread, crackers and other products should all be whole grain. Stay away from enriched wheat flour and items that claim "made with whole wheat flour". Very little is actually the whole grain.

Breads: Stay clear from anything white, and buy whole grain and sprouted grain. This goes for wraps as well.

Meat: Buy in bulk and divide the meat into servings once you are home. Look for lean cuts which are lower in saturated fat such as skinless chicken breast, extra lean ground beef, and of course your fish.

Condiments: Switch to low-fat dressings, mustards and mayonnaise. Marinades and bean spreads are also great to add flavour.

So now that you have all of your grocery shopping done, it is time to put them away. What is so great is that you already have a place for each and every item you have purchased. From here all you are doing is emptying the grocery store bins into your kitchen bins -it's quick and easy! This is a great way to have fun with the whole family and delegate so you can have family time while keeping the kitchen organized.

Personally, I like to pre-wash all of my veggies before they go into the fridge. I find that this saves me time throughout my busy week. I know where everything is and it's ready to go. I know it might seem like a lot at first, but it will save you a lot of stress as the week goes on! Kids love to help with this too - fill a sink with water and let them splash around!

Time to Cook

So, now that you have all of your food at home, it's time to cook! Cooking can be fun, creative and easy. I really suggest that over the next 13 weeks you try new things and be creative. Don't have the same old, same old every day. Liven it up a little. You can mix it up by changing your cooking methods, spices and or herbs or even what you want to add to the dish. Your options are endless. You can bake, broil, stir-fry, poach, grill, roast, sauté or steam your food. Use marinades and seasonings instead of frying your foods, have a fondue night and use a beef or chicken broth instead of oil.

Useful Kitchen Gadgets

Here are a few of the staples in my kitchen. I find that they not only save time, but they are fun to use:

- Non-stick frying pan – no need for fat when cooking
- Hand blender or regular blender - use for shakes and smoothies
- Mini food processor - blend veggies and add to dips
- A set of good knives - slicing and dicing
- Indoor grill - grill veggies and burgers
- Crockpot - it's great to have dinner ready when you come home
- Toaster oven - pop your sandwiches in for a real restaurant feel!
- Food dehydrator - fruit slices for snacks and salad toppings
- Cheese grater - shred some colourful veggies for decor on your dishes
- Garlic press - add fresh garlic to spice it up
- Melon baller - mini meatballs or even fruit kabobs

Conscious Eating

Meal times should be a time where you enjoy the food that you have created for you and your family. This is a time when we can truly be present with our bodies and feel proud of ourselves for the nourishment we are providing. I know we are all very busy, but let yourself take even one meal a day to sit down and pay attention to not only what you are eating but how it makes you feel.

Set the tone, sit at the dinner table and enjoy the dialogue with your family. Use place mats, napkins; use both the knife and fork while eating. Sure, light some candles, set the stage and enjoy your new Nutritional Lifestyle! Meal times are also a great way to lead by example if you have children. Being conscious and respectful of eating will teach them to live the same way.

"Nutritional Lifestyle" Tips

Don't let negative thoughts like, "I don't have time" or "It's too complicated" limit your success in this program. Empower yourself by taking control of your "Nutritional Lifestyle" with these tips.

- Have an organized fridge.
- Wash produce thoroughly as soon as you get home from the store, so it's ready when you need it.
- Prep your veggies for the week.
- Prep your veggies for each meal.
- Make bigger dinners and eat leftovers for lunch the next day.
- Prepare your lunches the night before.
- On the weekends, cook in bulk for the rest of the week.
- Freeze pancakes and put them in the toaster for a quick breakfast.
- Take bins or reusable bags to the grocery store to use for each food group.
- Freeze pasta sauce or chili in single serving plastic bags to defrost when you're ready.
- Stick a weekly meal planner on your fridge with meal plans and ingredients you'll need.
- Spices and herbs can transform any dish. Try out a new spice/herb each week.
- Try a night where your kids and spouse cook together.

Kids' Favourite

I wanted to add a little section here for our children. Many of you know that kids can be very fussy. You plan and make this wonderful meal only to have your children respond, "Oh I don't like that" or "Ew! What is that?!"

I've had to get creative in order for my daughter to establish her own healthy, fun and creative meals. Here's my way to "Fancy It Up".

"Fancy It Up" I find that when things look good and creative, kids feel special and excited to eat. Fancy it up by trying a few of these tricks:
- Try serving chopped veggies standing in a glass cup
- Serve yogurt in a fancy wine glass
- Fancy up the edge of a glass with a slice of fruit
- Sprinkle a little cocoa and icing sugar on a plate when you serve fresh fruit
- Freeze fresh yogurt in cones
- Cook pancakes into fun shapes. Use cookie cutters and get your kids to pick out which ones they want to use (just remember to spray with cooking spray)
- Place a little note in their lunch bags; just a few words that will let them know how special they are. We all need to be reminded sometimes!

Weekly Meals

I know what it's like to have a family on the go - you might not always think you have time for a nutritious lunch the next day. The good news is that you can use dinner to save you some time the next day! Dinners can become great lunches, quickly. Here are a few ways dinner can be transformed into lunch:

Sunday's rotisserie chicken can become a great chicken wrap for Monday's lunch. Take some chicken pieces and roll in a whole-wheat tortilla with a little Caesar dressing and some lettuce - lunch in seconds.

Cook extra chicken fingers and slice them. The next day, make a salad with the chicken finger slices, lettuce or spinach and any of your favourite salad toppings (nuts, seeds, veggies, etc). Just be sure to put your low-fat dressing in a separate container if you're taking it to work.

Have extra meatballs? Make a meat sauce by breaking up the meatballs and adding spaghetti sauce and green onion. Use as a dipping sauce for baked pita chips.

Chili is great to have for lunch the next day. For a change, place the leftover chili in a pita with grated cheese and green onions. Toast and serve with fat-free sour cream.

You don't need to be defeated by time limitations! Just plan ahead the night before and you will have quick and easy lunches the next day.

Weekly Meal Plan

MONDAY Carb: Protein: Fat:	Breakfast	Snack	Lunch	Snack	Dinner	Snack
TUESDAY Carb: Protein: Fat:	Breakfast	Snack	Lunch	Snack	Dinner	Snack
WEDNESDAY Carb: Protein: Fat:	Breakfast	Snack	Lunch	Snack	Dinner	Snack
THURSDAY Carb: Protein: Fat:	Breakfast	Snack	Lunch	Snack	Dinner	Snack
FRIDAY Carb: Protein: Fat:	Breakfast	Snack	Lunch	Snack	Dinner	Snack
SATURDAY Carb: Protein: Fat:	Breakfast	Snack	Lunch	Snack	Dinner	Snack
SUNDAY Carb: Protein: Fat:	Breakfast	Snack	Lunch	Snack	Dinner	Snack

liv

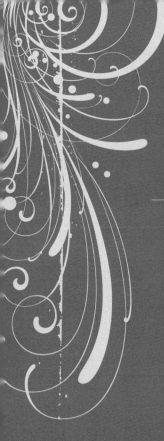

Be Forgiveness, where there is Forgiveness there is Peace and where there is Peace there is LOVE

Body & Exercise

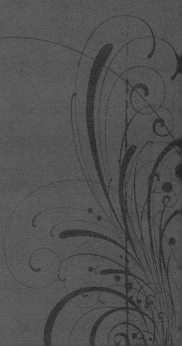

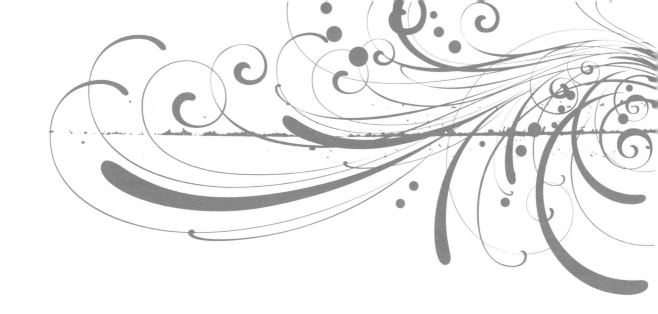

Chapter Ten
RELEASE YOUR INNER ATHLETE

"Movement is a medicine for creating change in a person's physical, emotional, and mental states."

Carol Welch

RELEASE YOUR INNER ATHLETE

I believe that within every one of us is an inner athlete waiting to shine. I have seen it, not only within myself but also with so many of my clients. There is an energy that is deep within us waiting to be unleashed, an energy that will completely transform your body and your life.

What separates the average person from the athlete is the state of control with their minds (and, yes, a little bit of genetics). However, if you were raised in a non-sports family like me, you may wonder how you could possibly be an athlete.

Before my transformation, I firmly believed it was all genetics. However, now I believe that each one of us has the ability to change, to tap into this unknown energy field and become that athlete.

I tell all of my clients that there are two ways you can work out - with your mind, or with your spirit. What's the difference, you might ask? When you work out with your mind, you might have thoughts that take over and have you rush through your sets and reps. You might become intimidated by your surroundings, or you might even give up and quit with only half of the completed sets. On the other hand, you might be thinking that you're indestructible and lift more than you should be. You are only using your attitude to try to manipulate your body.

Exercise has been around as long as humans. In the beginning, our exercise was running to - and from - our food. However, it wasn't until the early 18th century that exercise became tied to medicine and science. The world began to see aerobics, weight training and many exercises that we know today. It's also when the first fitness centres were opened. In the 19th century, the Industrial Revolution made life move faster and new health issues arose. It also saw the creation of fitness machines that people could use in their own homes, making exercise more accessible. Nowadays, exercise is everywhere - and confusing to most of us.

Working out with your spirit is completely different. It's funny, when I tell most of my clients this; they think I'm crazy until they actually feel the difference. When you begin any of your workouts, I encourage you to set the intention to remain focused, to feel your whole body when you enter this space. This means you should remain present, feel your breath, feel your joints moving and visualize your muscles becoming stronger with each rep. Be within your body and not your mind. Feel your increased vitality. When you do this, you cross the abyss into the energy of your inner athlete.

84

If you're looking for a quick fix, this is not it. You must be ready to finally own the body you live in. I explain it like this to all of my clients: it's like cleaning your house. Just one room at a time and then, all of a sudden you can start to see through the mess. This is the same. It takes a few weeks, but soon you will really begin to see the progress you're making. You might even find yourself, as I did, looking in the mirror every morning to see the changes happening. It was like Christmas every day!

Before you begin the exercise regime of the program, I want you to think about everything that your body does for you. I believe the more respect and attention we can give our bodies, the more it will repay us in wonderful ways.

Next in this section, I will review everything you need to know about your body, how it works and some fun and interesting facts about the bodies that we live in.

About our Bodies

Our physical bodies are truly unique. Each and every person is made up of 206 bones and more than 650 muscles. Our brain controls every aspect of our body, from growth to temperature to emotions. Our heart sends oxygen and nutrient-rich blood through our body and carries away the waste. Our digestive system breaks down food for absorption into the body. Our respiratory system helps us breathe without us even thinking about it. Our hormones affect the cells within our body, the immune system and reproduction system.

Your body is amazing! Imagine all the different activities that are occurring inside your body right now without you even noticing. Imagine the hundreds of reactions that take place inside your body to heal a broken bone, or how your body fights off a cold. When we eat, we engage our salivary glands, our tongue, our taste buds, our jaw muscles - and that's all before we even swallow our food! Just think of how awe-inspiring the simple process of digestion is. Our bodies just know what to do with almost anything that goes into our stomachs, even if we've never eaten it before. The body knows how to extract vitamins and minerals and transport them to the different organs, muscles and tissues that need them. It knows where to distribute energy. It knows what isn't useful for our bodies, and it sends it right out. As humans, we wouldn't even know where to start if we wanted to replicate something like that. It is so incredible!

Our bodies require care, and need a complete balance of exercise to strengthen our bones, muscles and joints, to maintain our weight, and to give us energy. But this also gives us the mentality to fully function and feel great about ourselves.

Are you helping your body out? Are you getting enough rest? Are you taking responsibility to ensure its strength and flexibility? You are the only one responsible for your body and I believe that we can use our physical body as a tool to strengthen the mind and ignite the spirit. I believe that the stronger we can become with our minds, the stronger we can become physically.

Common Excuses to Not Exercise

We've all heard the saying, "The road to hell is paved with good intentions." It's harsh, but it often rings true when it comes to exercise. We all have good intentions but our follow-through could use some work. Many people begin exercise routines but lose heart and give up partway through. Why is this? I find too many people allow their own self-talk to discourage them from their actual goal. It is then very easy for the mind to overcompensate and let you give into thoughts like, "I'm tired" or "I don't have time" - and then that's it. Your window of opportunity is gone. The biggest challenge in "The Ticket" is not the physical component as much as the mind steering you away from your goal. Remove these barriers of perception and you'll find exercise isn't quite so difficult after all!

"I have no time to exercise."
You don't need to spend hours at the gym to receive the benefits of exercise. Even 20 minutes of intense exercise is better than nothing at all. Break it up in 10-minute chunks throughout the day if it suits your schedule. As well, by missing out on the exercise, you are losing the benefits exercise has on your mind and spirit as well.

"I don't have equipment or a gym membership."
Save your money - you don't need a gym membership to work out. There are many exercises you can do at home with no or minimal equipment. If you have stairs, a counter and a chair, you can do squats, push-ups, tricep dips and step-ups. I designed the exercise library in this book to make it easy for you to get results with hardly any equipment needed.

"I have an injury or health condition that makes exercise difficult."
It takes exercise to strengthen your body. There is always some sort of exercise you can do without stressing the area of pain or worsening a health issue. Your body is a reflection of how you treat it - chronic injuries or conditions can be prevented from worsening or improve with exercise. Ease into the program and you may find that you continue to gain strength.

"Exercise takes too long and there are products I can buy that save time."
There are no easy fixes. Your body needs real exercise to achieve cardiovascular health and to build muscle and flexibility. You need to work your muscles, not just shake or rotate them. Concentrating on your exercise, being present in your thoughts and actions will help you transform yourself through your commitment.

"I just want to lose weight, so I need cardio."
Cardio exercises are great for your health, but they're not the only way to lose weight. The more muscle you have, the higher your metabolism and therefore the more calories you burn. Include strength training in your workout regime.

"I'm a woman, I don't want to strength train and look like a bodybuilder."
It's not physically possible for everyday women to become as muscular as female bodybuilders without the aid of supplements and endless hours at the gym. Working out isn't about how big your muscles are or the six-pack. It's about owning your own inner strength and then reflecting it back at you in your own physical body.

"Working out is boring."
It doesn't have to be. These are just your past thoughts. With "The Ticket", your exercise time is your time to dream, create and become engaged with your life. Be excited for yourself - you're finding your inner power!

Components of Fitness

Your workout regime should consist of a balance of cardio, strength training and flexibility elements. Here's a bit of information about all three.

Cardio: Cardiovascular exercise (aerobic exercise) is any form of movement that increases your heart rate. Cardio exercise is one of the greatest anti-aging treatments available to anyone: muscle and strength gain, loss of fat, increased energy, greater wellbeing and a decrease in anxiety and depression. Moreover, aerobic exercise also lowers blood pressure, improves the immune system and helps protect the body against a host of diseases, including cardiovascular diseases, stroke, hypertension, diabetes, and osteoporosis.

Strength Training: No matter what your fitness goals, strength training is vital. It helps to prevent osteoporosis, builds lean muscle and increases your metabolism so you can burn fat. Here is your chance to prove to yourself how strong you really are. Build your muscles to reflect on that inner courage, strength and power!

Flexibility: Stretching helps to keep your muscles limber, increase your flexibility and allows yourself time to reflect on your workout. In the last five to ten minutes of your workout, use your stretching time to bring yourself back into awareness with your body. Listen to your soundtrack and think about where you want to go in your life. Make sure you stretch every muscle group you worked out. Hold stretches for 20 to 30 seconds and don't bounce or jerk. You shouldn't feel any pain - it should feel good!

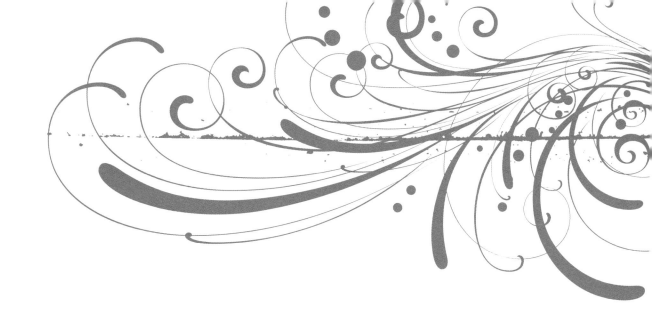

Chapter Eleven
LET'S GET STARTED!

"It is exercise alone that supports the spirits,
and keeps the mind in vigor."

Marcus Tullius Cicero

LET'S GET STARTED

This section is where you'll learn all that is needed to know about exercise. Don't feel discouraged if you don't know what some of the terms mean - they're all explained in this chapter. We'll also cover the information that you'll need to keep in mind while exercising, how to monitor your heart rate and know where to start.

Fitness Levels

This book will provide a variety of exercises for every fitness level. Here is how to tell which level you're in:

BRONZE: You have no experience with an exercise program or haven't worked out. You are someone who wants to ease into the program. You may have limited your cardiovascular exercise to walking. You're not use to a raised and consistent heart rate. You may have health problems. If you're a bronze, don't be discouraged by this new exercise regime - be excited! Be proud of yourself that you have taken the initiative to become stronger. Don't push yourself too hard and don't lose heart. Your body is going to be adapting quickly over the next 13 weeks, so take it one day at a time.

SILVER: You are working out three to five times a week. You can do cardio for at least 20 minutes. You're someone who is looking to take your fitness to the next level. Since you do have some exercise experience, you may feel you are not seeing any results. Don't give up! Use this chance to mix it up when you're exercising and try new things. Feel the power of your mind and have positive thoughts to advance yourself!

GOLD: You can run for a minimum of 30 minutes and are used to high-intensity workouts. You're in good shape, but are looking for the next challenge. With this program, you're going to take your fitness to the next level. Let yourself tune into your body and listen to what it needs. If you've been working out for a few years, you may be surprised that your body wants more rest than it gets, or it wants to try different things than you expect. Just embrace the journey and have fun!

Every four weeks your body should be stressed so it can be healed and become stronger. This means you should increase the intensity or scope of your workouts monthly. It might be the only time in your life that stress is good for you!

With a balanced exercise program, you need a cardio component, a strength component and a flexibility component. All three are very important in each workout. And, as with every new thing you try, don't be embarrassed of how much you can or can't do at the beginning. We all started with 10-minute power walks or five-pound weights! The key is to keep at it and let the power inside you grow.

Fitness Gauge

The Fitness Gauge is designed to test your core, upper and lower body strength as well as your cardiovascular strength. This is a gauge that you will be using four times throughout the next 84 days: now and after the completion of weeks 4, 8 and 12. This will be the benchmark for you to see the results from hard work and dedication to your workouts.

You will perform your gauge on the same day you complete your measurements. Please don't allow yourself to be intimidated as this is just for you to use as a tool to see and celebrate your progress. Have fun with it! You may find it difficult now but I promise you that as time goes on, you will become more excited to do this test. Here are the simple exercises that you will perform in the Fitness Gauge test.

A few reminders:
- Depending on your level: Bronze, Silver or Gold, you will perform the same exercises each time, with only a few modifications. You can find your fitness level on page 90.
- Remember to keep track of your starting position so you can see your progress.
- Be sure to check out proper techniques for each exercise found in the exercise library.
- Perform a few reps of each exercise by itself. This will also ensure that you are familiar with how to perform each one!
- Don't forget to mark your time and your HR.

Exercises:
- **Upper Body**: Push-ups *(page 187)*
- **Lower Body:** Squats *(page 174)*
- **Core:** Sit-ups *(page 212)*
- **Cardio:** Walking or running

- Bronze: 10 reps
- Silver: 15 reps
- Gold: 25 reps

These exercises are to be completed around the perimeter of a small soccer field, a baseball park, a park or a large enough backyard. Your chosen space should be either square or rectangular in shape. Make sure you time yourself and take your heart rate when you're done.

1. Start with a warm up, like walking around and performing a few reps of each exercise.

2. When ready, run to one corner of the space.

3. Complete push-ups here.

4. Get up and run to the corner of the space to your left.

5. Complete sit-ups here.

6. Get up and run to the next corner to your left.

7. Complete squats here.

8. Sprint back to the corner where you started.

Level: BRONZE (10 reps)

Starting Point:_____   Time:_____   Heart Rate:_____
Week 4:_____   Time:_____   Heart Rate:_____
Week 8:_____   Time:_____   Heart Rate:_____
Week 12:_____   Time:_____   Heart Rate:_____

Level: SILVER (15 reps)

Starting Point:_____   Time:_____   Heart Rate:_____
Week 4:_____   Time:_____   Heart Rate:_____
Week 8:_____   Time:_____   Heart Rate:_____
Week 12:_____   Time:_____   Heart Rate:_____

Level: GOLD (25 reps)

Starting Point:_____   Time:_____   Heart Rate:_____
Week 4:_____   Time:_____   Heart Rate:_____
Week 8:_____   Time:_____   Heart Rate:_____
Week 12:_____   Time:_____   Heart Rate:_____

I always like to consider these benchmark days as celebration days. You need to take a break from time to time and look back to see the progress you have made, and that's where this fitness gauge comes in.

Sets and Reps

"Rep" is short for repetition, and refers to the amount of times you perform the same action in a row, such as raising and lowering a weight or doing a push-up. Sets are the amount of reps done in a row. Sets are separated by an amount of time called a rest. The basic level is two to three sets of 12.

Rest

A rest is a pause between your sets and reps. The most common is 30 seconds to one minute between reps and one to two minutes between sets.

Fitness Principles

No matter whether you are Bronze, Silver or Gold, you will probably want some level of control over your workout routines. Here are some of the principles The Ticket exercises are based on. Use these principles to help you design your own workout routines.

FITNESS LEVEL	FREQUENCY (days per week) *Ensure you allow at least one day of rest per week	DURATION	CARDIO Intensity (HR Range)	STRENGTH Sets, Reps, & Rest
Bronze:	Cardio: 3-4 Strength: 2-3 Flexibility: 4-7	Cardio: 20-30 mins Strength: 20-30 mins Flexibility: 10 mins	Low End: 55-65% High End: 64-75%	Sets: 2-3 Reps: 8-12 Rest: 30-90 sec
Silver:	Cardio: 3-4 Strength: 2-3 Flexibility: 4-7	Cardio: 30-40 mins Strength: 35-40 mins Flexibility: 10 mins	Low End: 55-65% High End: 70-80%	Sets: 2-3 Reps: 10-15 Rest: 30-90 sec
Gold:	Cardio: 3-4 Strength: 2-3 Flexibility: 4-7	Cardio: up to 60 mins Strength: 30-45 mins Flexibility: 10 mins	Low End: 60-75% High End: 80-95%	Sets: 3-4 Reps: 15-25 Rest: as needed

*Adequate rest is crucial for the body to repair itself. Ensure you allow 36-48 hrs rest for muscles/groups worked to repair. *For example: If you strength train your lower body on Monday wait at least until Wednesday or Thursday to train them again. Use Tuesday as a cardio or upper body workout. See Program sections for example*

Types of Programs

Aside from the basic sets and reps for each exercise, you can use these additional programs to add some spice to your routines!

Circuit: Circuit training develops strength, flexibility, cardiovascular health, coordination and endurance at the same time. It consists of a wide variety of short exercises in one session, with a minimal amount of rest.

Interval: Interval training is exercise that consists of spurts of high-energy activity alternated with low intensity or rest. An example of interval training is a period of sprinting followed by a period of slow jogging, and so on.

Pyramid: Pyramid training is where you perform the reps as follows: 12-10-8-10-12, meaning there would be five different sets.

Super sets: Super sets are two different exercises for one particular muscle or group. For example, try doing a set of lunges then super setting with a set of squats, or a chest press followed by push-ups.

Heart Rate

Your heart rate is going to be the most important tool for you to use through this program. Throughout the program, you'll be using your heart rate as your tangible indication for your workout intensity. This is a tangible gauge to show you your increase in cardiovascular strength.

Resting Heart Rate (RHR): Your resting heart rate is your HR, when your body isn't undertaking any activity. To figure out your resting heart rate, count your heartbeats for one minute as soon as you wake up while still resting in bed. Try to get your resting HR on days that you do not need the alarm to get you up. Do this for three consecutive mornings. Divide these three numbers by three to give you an average for your resting heart rate.

Maximum Heart Rate (MHR): The maximum heart rate is the highest rate your heart can safely beat per minute. You can find your maximum heart rate by subtracting your age from 220 for males and 226 for females.

Your Target Heart Rate: depends on your level of fitness. Exercising in this range will give your cardiovascular system the best workout. It's approximately 55% - 90% of your maximum heart rate. Beginners, of course, should try not to be superheroes and push themselves to 90%. Stay within the intensity that's right for you and move up, as you progress.

Females:
(226 - age) = MHR - (RHR x %) + RHR =_____

Males:
(220 - age) = MHR - (RHR x %) + RHR = _____

liv

Heart Rate Monitors: You will need to monitor your heart rate during your workouts. You can do it the old-fashioned way by finding your pulse, or I suggest you purchase a heart rate monitor. There are a variety of heart rate monitors to choose from. Monitors are combined with watches; some are in two pieces - a watch with a band that goes around your chest.

Exercise Scale: The other gauge I like to use is called the "Exercise Scale." I have used this scale with all of my clients as we all start at different levels. Here, you are going to create a measure of your endurance from one to ten.

- One is at the bottom of the scale where you are sitting on the couch doing nothing.

- Five is where you are beginning to move and feel your blood pumping. You should be feeling like you are getting a bit of a workout.

- Seven is where your heart rate is up there. You're feeling it and you begin to have thoughts that you want to slow down or even quit.

- Nine to 10 is where you (safely) push through your mind barriers and begin to flow with your spirit. You feel free, light and completely filled with power and strength.

Posture

My favourite quote for a long time has been: ***"You can or you can't and either way you are right."*** by Henry Ford.

This is so true, as our attitude and posture go hand in hand with the success of your program. If you allow your negative self to defeat you then this is the result you are going to have. However, if you approach things with an *I can* attitude, then you know what? You *can*! So if you want to feel empowered in your life, taking control becomes first and foremost from the attitude with which we carry ourselves.

For as long as I remember I always wanted to have good posture. I remember looking at my wedding pictures and wondered why I was always hunched over with rounded shoulders and my head was so far out there. Even after the birth of my daughter I always caught myself looking in the mirror and trying to stand up straight, with proper alignment.

I believe that the more you take ownership of your life, even in small ways, the more you will notice your posture change. From here you will then be able to see yourself standing straight and walking tall. It was not until after my transformation that I was finally able to own my whole self and be proud of who I am. Then it seemed that my posture shifted to reflect this new energy shift within me.

With exercise, posture is extremely important as well. Having a strong foundation will not only empower you in your routine, but it will also prevent injury.

INCORRECT POSTURE:

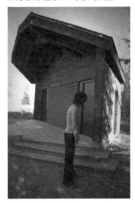

Here is how the body should be aligned. Start with your feet. Looking down, align yourself so your ankles are in line with your knees and your knees are in line with your hips. Your hips should be in line with your shoulders, and your shoulders should be in line with your ears, your chest should be tall, your shoulders back, and your core tight.

Try this test to check and feel proper posture. Stand with your arms at 45 degrees and place a broom handle horizontally through the space between your elbows and your back, your chest should rise and your shoulders are back. This is what I call **POSTURE**. Walk around your house for a few minutes a day. It will help you stay straight!

CORRECT POSTURE:

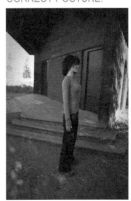

If you like, you can have someone evaluate your posture for you, or take a look in a full-length mirror. Try looking at your posture when you aren't thinking about it, like when you're walking outside past a tall window. Don't judge, just observe.

An excellent exercise to help build the muscles for improving your posture is the Wall Angel found on page 197.

liv

Equipment:

I have designed this program to use as little equipment as possible. This way, you'll be able to take your exercise routine anywhere you go.

Running shoes: Invest in good shoes. Even if you don't do high-impact exercises, you don't want to take risks with your spine and joints. Go to an athletic or running store and get someone to help you. Trust the experts and don't be too turned off by the price tag - don't break the bank, but do buy shoes that will support you and last for a long time.

Heart rate monitor: You have read about heart rate monitors earlier in the chapter, now spend some time searching for the one that works for you. It should be comfortable and user-friendly.

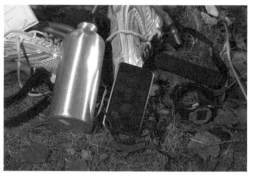

MP3 Player: Music is essential to keep you interested and having fun. Look for a music player that has a clip or holder you can attach to your clothes. You can listen to any music you prefer, but make sure you don't have the volume too loud. Especially if you're exercising outside, stay safe and make sure you can hear the world around you. Don't feel like you need to splurge on a fancy music player, but remember, your soundtrack is part of your motivation for your challenge.

Water bottle: Get a good water bottle! You need your water, so don't cheap out. Get one that doesn't leak, doesn't slip and, if possible, has an attachment you can use to secure it to your clothing.

Resistance band: A resistance band is a stretchy cord or band with handles on either end. It helps you with certain stretches or exercises by providing resistance. You can find these in many places, such as your local department store or any athletic store. You can purchase bands with different resistance as well as removable handles. These are the ones that I suggest - as you progress you're going to need to increase your resistance, and your upper and lower body will also require a different intensity.

Breathing

Breathing is essential for you to live, and it's essential in exercising as well. Our breath is what carries the oxygen to the muscles for strength. Start with a deep cleansing breath, breathing from your diaphragm and feeling the oxygen fill your chest cavity. When performing a movement in exercise, exhale upon the exertion.

Drink Your Water

Water is essential for our survival. It lubricates our joints, assists in the transportation of nutrients and helps eliminate waste. It is the main ingredient of all body fluids and is involved in every single bodily function.

A good rule of thumb is half your weight in pounds is the number of ounces your body requires to function optimally. For example, a 130 lbs. woman needs 65 oz. of water per day, or 8 x 8 oz. cups. Or just look at the colour of your urine. If your urine is a light yellow to a clear colour, you know you're getting enough water.

Drinking water while exercising is especially crucial. It helps to replace the fluid leaving your body when you perspire, hydrates your muscles and prevents overheating.

Tips for Exercising

- Use this time for yourself. Create the time, the intention, and be present in the moment. Don't rush.

- Use your REAL Motivation cards while working out to make sure you're feeling everything and your mind isn't wandering. Use this to help you bring your spirit and mind into your exercise.

- Use your power words with every inhale and exhale.

- Visualize.

- Put your heart and soul into your exercise.

- Drink lots of water while exercising.

- Make sure you know what exercises and program you're going to be doing each week.

- Find music to exercise to that makes you feel empowered.

- Exercise first thing in the morning. Not only does it start up the motor of your body, but it prevents excuses. You feel so good about getting it done that your energy is high all day.

- Start with a warm up to get the blood flowing. Normally, a warm up is cardio for five to 10 minutes. It's a good idea to warm up the muscles you plan to exercise that day.

- Next, move on to strength training and finally to flexibility.

- In your strength training, pay attention to the muscle you're working in each rep. Make sure you can feel it.

- Take time to pause between each individual exercise. The length of this pause depends on your fitness level.

- Make sure you breathe. Exhale on exertion and inhale on the easiest movement.

- Rest between sets.

- Prepare your mind to get ready for the next rep.

- In strength training, you will know you are at the right weight level when the last rep or two feels difficult, but still manageable. You want to push yourself, but within safe limits.

- Remember to cool down after your workout. Reflect on how present you felt while exercising. Were you rushing to get through it, or were you being present and feeling your own strength? Use your stretching cool down time to relax and reflect back on your workout, prepare yourself for your day and get excited about your life.

As with anything, I believe quality is better than quantity. Don't be concerned with how many exercises you can do. Concentrate on putting your full effort into each one. This is when the true magnitude of your strength will be revealed. Use your REAL Motivation card and your affirmations to remind yourself why you're doing this and I bet you'll find you have the energy to run up that hill or run that last kilometer.

The best part of this program is that you will be able to see and feel your inner strength transform into your outer physical strength. No matter where you are along your exercise path, all that matters is that you're willing to show to yourself what you are actually capable of achieving.

Your Measurements

Taking measurements is a tangible way to see your body transform from your hard work. You will be taking your measurements 4 times through the next 13 weeks: now, and at the end of week 4, 8 and 12.

Make these benchmark days a Celebration. I suggest completing your measurements the same day as your Fitness Gauge. (Page 91)

It is best to have the same person or yourself do your measurements. The mirror is an excellent guide to ensure you measure in the same place each time. Measure the following areas:

- Right arm
- Chest (nipple line)
- High waist (the smallest part of your waist)
- Belly button (where your belly button is)
- Hips (the widest part of your buttocks)
- Right thigh (the largest part of your thigh)

Date: _____ (week 0)
Starting Weight: _____
Right Arm: _____
Chest: _____
High Waist: _____
Belly Button: _____
Hips: _____
Thigh: _____

HOW YOUR BODY

INSPIRES YOUR LIFE

STRONG LOWER BODY: A strong lower body is a strong foundation. Feel the power and strength drawn from this area of your body.

CORE: Your core is the centre of your body, home of your heart, chest and vital organs. Feel and own your enthusiasm, your creativity and your confidence that stems from this section of your body that is full of life.

BACK & SHOULDERS: Stand tall, straight and proud. Own your presence and let your true personality shine through.

Your Ultimate Body

Week 4
Weight: _____
Right Arm: _____
Chest: _____
High Waist: _____
Belly Button: _____
Hips: _____
Thigh: _____

Week 8
Weight: _____
Right Arm: _____
Chest: _____
High Waist: _____
Belly Button: _____
Hips: _____
Thigh: _____

Week 12
Weight: _____
Right Arm: _____
Chest: _____
High Waist: _____
Belly Button: _____
Hips: _____
Thigh: _____

Flip through a variety of
magazines and find your
ultimate body

Glue your
Ultimate
Body here.

Now that you've taken your measurements and you have your starting weight, hide the scale. Have someone else hide it if you need too! The temptation to constantly weigh yourself can become compulsive. Have faith and trust that you are moving closer to your goal each day. I will never forget my eighth week when I weighed myself. I was down to 136 pounds, which I had not weighed for years. The more you allow yourself to follow with trust and faith, the easier your body changes and adapts.

I suggest you take a picture of yourself at the beginning of this transformation as a visual reminder of your starting point. It's so amazing to compare this before picture to your Celebration pictures when you complete the 13 weeks (pg.164). Wear what you feel most comfortable in, maybe it's a fitted tank top with shorts, or a two-piece bathing suit. Either way, this picture will be a visual reminder of how the body follows where the mind and spirit lead it.

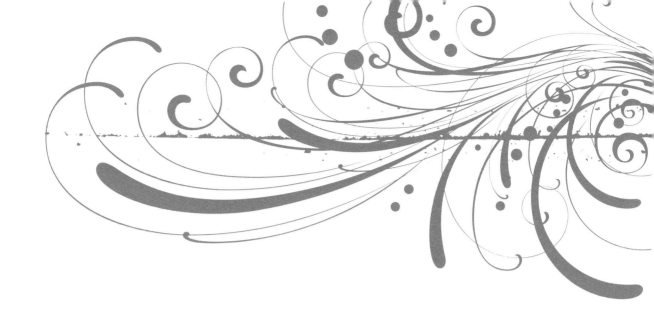

Chapter Twelve
OWNING YOUR WORKOUTS

"The five S's of sports training are: stamina, speed, strength, skill, and spirit; but the greatest of these is spirit."

Ken Doherty

OWNING YOUR WORKOUTS

Working Out

This is where you get a chance to give it your all. This means pushing yourself to achieve whatever it is that you want in this life. The more you push your physical body, the more you will uncover the strength to achieve your REAL Motivation.

Trust me, your mind will always try to come up with excuses as to why you can't keep to your workouts or make you think you don't have time. You are stronger than that! I believe that each one of us deserves to look in the mirror and see a body that we are proud to have. We should all be able to walk down the street with our heads held high, our shoulders back and have a presence that radiates from within us. You can give yourself this gift, and it starts now.

The exercise program in this section consists of your basic exercises, with a few variations added to change them up at each level. You'll be amazed how quickly you will see your body become stronger. When I started at the beginning, I couldn't even do a push up or a sit up let alone even trying to attempt a "burpie." Just keep with it. As you begin to own your spirit, your mind and your body will follow!

This program is for you, and no one else. While you may choose to workout with a buddy or a partner, I recommend that you take this time for you and you alone. Get to know yourself. Realize how close your dreams are, and create the life that you always envisioned.

Where should you work out? I encourage you to go outside and fill your body with fresh air. There is nothing more refreshing for your mind, body and your spirit. Don't be afraid to go outside in the winter either – there is always something you can do! These exercises can be completed anywhere. The only equipment you need is your shoes, your music, your REAL Motivation Card, your heart rate monitor and your resistance band. However, if you feel more comfortable using other equipment such as weights - go for it. Work out where you feel most comfortable, where you will be able to relax and have this time with yourself.

Things to Remember

- Don't rush it! Enjoy each step. Enjoy the strength that you gain with each and every workout. As long as you take it day by day you will make it to the finish line, I promise!

- Work out first thing in the morning. It might be a little hard at first, but with your REAL Motiviation you will be energized for the rest of the day. You won't have any excuses later in the day if you work out as soon as you wake up! And, yes, you can work out in your pyjamas - as long as you do it!

- Visualize the muscles becoming stronger. Place your attention on your muscle or group that you are training.

- When lifting, contract your abdominal muscles, make sure you lift through your legs and not your back. Bring your attention to your abs and squeeze them. Really concentrate on this the first few times so you know what it feels like and you know you're doing it properly.

- Keep your core tight as it provides stability, and also supports the lower back. This is just a slight tightening of the abdominals. Here is a little exercise that might help. Lie on your back and place your fingers on the inside of your hipbones. Pretend to cough and feel how slightly your core activates.

- Posture: Head, shoulders and hips should be in alignment (refer to page 97).

- Try not to 'lock' joints while performing an exercise.

- Keep knees and ankles aligned where possible. Knees should not go over toes

- Breathe! Sometimes we get so caught up in things that we forget about our breathing. Always inhale on starting position and exhale on the exertion. Just do the best you can and as each workout progresses you'll see your form and breathing techniques fall into place.

- Always warm up for five to 10 minutes to get the blood flowing. Move, increase your heart rate, warm up those joints, and the muscles that you will be working. You can even do a few repetitions of that particular exercise in your warm-up as well. Use this time to get prepared for your workout.

- Always cool down; depending on the level of intensity a cool down can involve a slow jog, or walking, It's important to allow your heart rate to slowly return to the lower end of your scale. Take 5-10 minutes at the end of your cardio session while decreasing your intensity level to ensure your HR lowers at an even pace.

- It's important to stretch the muscles you have worked. This will help aid their repair, which may alleviate the delayed muscle soreness felt after training. Flexibility training also helps to strengthen and lengthen the muscles and joints.

- Stop if you feel any sharp pains, dizziness, nausea or difficulty breathing.

This is where you get to bring the REAL Motivation into practice and harness your power to create your best life. This is the time to make yourself the biggest priority in your life. No one but you can change your life!

Program Examples

In this section, I have designed three different programs for each level: Bronze, Silver and Gold. If you stick with this, you will be able to grow in body, mind and spirit.

These are only examples of what a program may look like for each level, but your options are limitless. Focus on having a new outlook and trying something new. Push yourself a little, listen to your inner guide, and most of all have fun! Use these exercises as the basis of a balanced program and find what works for you!

BRONZE
Program 1

"Down in the Basement" (Bronze P1) is designed to build a base or foundation. In order to build a house you need to start with a good foundation. This is the purpose in Bronze P1. This is a full body strength training program, with cardio sessions on alternating days.. This is the initial step in building your foundation in all three components of fitness; Strength, Cardiovascular and Flexibility.

The strength training component of this is program is designed to be completed in your basement, the cardio component, outside. However, feel free to change the locations for either.

Schedule

	Monday	Tuesday	Wednesday	Thursday	Friday	Saturday	Sunday
Week 1	**Strength:** *Full Body* *reps: 8 sets: 2* Flexibility:	**Cardio** *Walk:* *25-30 mins* Flexibility:	**Strength:** *Full Body or Rest* *reps: 8 sets: 2* Flexibility:	**Cardio** *Walk:* *25-30 mins* Flexibility:	**Strength:** *Full Body* *reps: 8 sets: 2* Flexibility:	**Cardio or Rest** *Walk:* *25-30 mins* Flexibility:	Rest
Week 2	**Strength:** *Full Body* *reps: 10 sets: 2* Flexibility:	**Cardio** *Walk:* *25-30 mins* Flexibility:	**Strength:** *Full Body or Rest* *reps: 10 sets: 2* Flexibility:	**Cardio** *Walk:* *25-30 mins* Flexibility:	**Strength:** *Full Body* *reps: 10 sets: 2* Flexibility:	**Cardio or Rest** *Walk:* *25-30 mins* Flexibility:	Rest
Week 3	**Strength:** *Full Body* *reps: 8 sets: 3* Flexibility:	**Cardio** *Walk:* *30-35 mins* Flexibility:	**Strength:** *Full Body or Rest* *reps: 8 sets: 3* Flexibility:	**Cardio** *Walk:* *30-35 mins* Flexibility:	**Strength:** *Full Body* *reps: 8 sets: 3* Flexibility:	**Cardio** *Walk:* *30-35 mins* Flexibility:	Rest
Week 4	**Strength:** *Full Body* *reps: 10 sets: 3* Flexibility:	**Cardio** *Walk:* *30-35 mins* Flexibility:	**Strength:** *Full Body or Rest* *reps: 10 sets: 3* Flexibility:	**Cardio** *Walk:* *30-35 mins* Flexibility:	**Strength:** *Full Body* *reps: 10 sets: 3* Flexibility:	**Cardio** *Walk:* *30-35 mins* Flexibility:	Rest

liv

Cardio: *"The Walk"* Walking is the best activity to start when engaging in a Cardio program. A good rule of thumb, when setting your pace is to move as there is a purpose to your jaunt, not too fast and not too slow. Ground yourself and feel your breath entering and exiting your body.

Posture is important as well when walking, remember these points:
- Head straight, shoulders back, ears over shoulders
- Core is tight; chest is tall
- Upper body slightly leaning back
- Long lean stride; heel-toe action; and long deep breaths

You might even want to envision yourself pushing from the ground, or even squeezing your glutes with each stride.

Target Heart Rate: 55% - 70%

Strength Training: *"The Sets"* As you begin this program, just remember that we are building muscle. With each strength training session your body is becoming stronger and needs to be stressed even further to continue to increase strength. Each week increase either your number of reps or sets. For example:
- Week 1 (Reps: 8, Sets: 2)
- Week 2 (Reps: 10, Sets: 2)
- Week 3 (Reps: 8, Sets: 3)
- Week 4 (Reps: 10, Sets: 3)

Target Heart Rate: 55% - 65%

Flexibility: Gently stretch the muscles worked and any muscles that feel tight. Tune into your body and stretch accordingly. Remember to breathe deep from your diaphragm and hold each stretch for 30 - 60 seconds.

Don't push too hard at the very start and run the risk of injury. Allow yourself to progress naturally. This is a journey, allow it to unfold.

Workout

Bronze Program 1

'Down in the Basement'

Cardio/Warm-up:

Muscle	Exercise
Warm-up	5 - 10 minutes HR Target 55%
Cardio	Walking: See program HR targets and durations

Strength:

Muscle	Exercise		Reps	Sets	Rest
LOWER BODY					
Quad/Hamstring	Basic Lunge	pg. 170	8-10	2-3	30-90s
Glutes	Touch Squat	pg. 173	8-10	2-3	30-90s
Calves	Walking Calf Raises	pg. 185	8-10	2-3	30-90s
UPPER BODY					
Chest	Push-Ups (wall)	pg. 188	8-10	2-3	30-90s
Back	Seated Row	pg. 194	8-10	2-3	30-90s
CORE					
Abs	Basic Sit-up	pg. 212	8-10	2-3	30-90s
Upper	Basic Crunch	pg. 215	8-10	2-3	30-90s
Lower Back	Basic Superman	pg. 209	8-10	2-3	30-90s

Flexibility:

Muscle	Stretch		Hold	Sets
LOWER BODY				
Quad	Standing Quads Stretch	pg. 235	30-60s	1
Hamstring	Hamstring Stretch	pg. 235	30-60s	1
Glutes	Tree Glute Stretch	pg. 236	30-60s	1
Calves	Toes Up Stretch	pg. 235	30-60s	1
Thighs	Feet First Stretch	pg. 237	30-60s	1
UPPER BODY				
Chest	Tree Chest Stretch	pg. 238	30-60s	1
Shoulders	Shoulder Cross Stretch	pg. 239	30-60s	1
CORE				
Lower Back	Twist Glute Stretch	pg. 238	30-60s	1

liv

The objective of the first month of your program is to become in tune with your body. The more you are able to activate each muscle the stronger and faster you will begin to see your results. Learn to stay in the present by allowing your mind to only focus on each exercise and your muscles becoming stronger. It is your mind that leads and the body follows.

You will find that the Cardio component of your program becomes easier as your body gains efficiency in transporting oxygen to your cells. Your muscles are now becoming conditioned and you should be seeing your results.

BRONZE
Program 2

Schedule

In weeks 5-8 of this program you will be performing a split routine. Your full body routine is now two programs: a lower body and upper body.

	Monday	Tuesday	Wednesday	Thursday	Friday	Saturday	Sunday
Week 5	**Strength:** *Upper Body* *reps: 8 sets: 2*	**Cardio** *Walk:* *30-35 mins*	**Strength:** *Lower Body or Rest* *reps: 8 sets: 2*	**Cardio** *Walk:* *30-35 mins*	**Strength:** *Upper Body* *reps: 8 sets: 2*	**Cardio or Rest** *Walk:* *30-35 mins*	Rest
	Flexibility:	**Flexibility:**	**Flexibility:**	**Flexibility:**	**Flexibility:**	**Flexibility:**	
Week 6	**Strength:** *Lower Body* *reps: 10 sets: 2*	**Cardio** *Walk:* *30-35 mins*	**Strength:** *Upper Body or Rest* *reps: 10 sets: 2*	**Cardio** *Walk:* *30-35 mins*	**Strength:** *Lower Body* *reps: 10 sets: 2*	**Cardio** *Walk:* *30-35 mins*	Rest
	Flexibility:	**Flexibility:**	**Flexibility:**	**Flexibility:**	**Flexibility:**	**Flexibility:**	
Week 7	**Strength:** *Upper Body* *reps: 10 sets: 3*	**Cardio** *Walk:* *30-35 mins*	**Strength:** *Lower Body* *reps: 10 sets: 3*	**Cardio** *Walk:* *30-35 mins*	**Strength:** *Upper Body* *reps: 10 sets: 3*	**Cardio** *Walk:* *30-35 mins*	Rest
	Flexibility:	**Flexibility:**	**Flexibility:**	**Flexibility:**	**Flexibility:**	**Flexibility:**	
Week 8	**Strength:** *Lower Body* *reps: 12 sets: 3*	**Cardio** *Walk:* *30-35 mins*	**Strength:** *Upper Body* *reps: 12 sets: 3*	**Cardio** *Walk:* *30-35 mins*	**Strength:** *Lower Body* *reps: 12 sets: 3*	**Cardio** *Walk:* *30-35 mins*	Rest
	Flexibility:	**Flexibility:**	**Flexibility:**	**Flexibility:**	**Flexibility:**	**Flexibility:**	

Cardio: *"The Walk"* If you have been walking for your cardio days, it's time to increase your intensity in P2. Try a nearby park, some stairs or even a hill. Take your cardio to a new level by stopping at every bench and completing a few step-ups (pg 176), and watch your HR increase.

Target Heart Rate: 64% - 75%

liv

Strength Training: *"Out at the Park" "In the Kitchen"* The upper and lower body programs are designed for different locations. "Out at the Park" (P2a) is an upper body strength routine. You can add a little extra cardio time by choosing a park that is a little further away and walk/jog there as your warm up. "In the Kitchen" is the lower body strength routine that uses your furniture as your equipment. Sometimes it's nice to change the scenery, however if you prefer to use a park or your basement this is fine as well.

- Week 5 (Reps: 8, Sets: 2)
- Week 6 (Reps: 10, Sets: 2)
- Week 7 (Reps: 10, Sets: 3)
- Week 8 (Reps: 12, Sets: 3) **Target Heart Rate:** 55% - 65%

Flexibility: Gently stretch the muscles worked and any muscles that feel tight. Tune into your body and stretch accordingly. Remember to breathe deep from your diaphragm and hold each stretch for 30 - 60 seconds.

Workout
Bronze Program 2
'Out at the Park' (upper body)

Cardio/Warm-up:

Muscle	Exercise
Warm-up	5 - 10 minutes HR Target 55%
Cardio	Walking: See program HR targets and durations

Strength:

Muscle	Exercise		Reps	Sets	Rest
UPPER BODY					
Chest	Push-Ups (wall)	pg. 188	8-12	2-3	45s
Back	Seated Row	pg. 194	8-12	2-3	45s
Biceps	Basic Bicep Curls	pg. 206	8-12	2-3	45s
Triceps	Standing Triceps Extension	pg. 203	8-12	2-3	45s
Shoulders	Seated Earth Raiser	pg. 200	8-12	2-3	45s
CORE					
Lower	Basic V-twist	pg. 227	8-12	2-3	45s
Upper	Basic Sit-up	pg. 212	8-12	2-3	45s
Lower Back	Intermediate Superman	pg. 210	8-12	2-3	45s

Flexibility:

Muscle	Stretch		Hold	Sets
UPPER BODY				
Chest	Tree Chest Stretch	pg. 238	30-60s	1
Biceps	Thumbs Down Stretch	pg. 239	30-60s	1
Triceps	Overhead Triceps Stretch	pg. 239	30-60s	1
Shoulders	Shoulder Cross Stretch	pg. 239	30-60s	1
CORE				
Lower Back	Twist Glute Stretch	pg. 238	30-60s	1

Workout

Bronze Program 2

"In the Kitchen' (lower body)

Cardio/Warm-up:

Muscle	Exercise
Warm-up	5 - 10 minutes HR Target 55%
Cardio	Walking: See program HR targets and durations

Strength:

Muscle	Exercise		Reps	Sets	Rest
LOWER BODY					
Quad	Basic Lunge	pg. 170	8-12	2-3	45s
Hamstring	Basic One Legged Dip	pg. 179	8-12	2-3	45s
Glutes	Basic Bridge	pg. 182	8-12	2-3	45s
Calves	Walking Calf Raises	pg. 185	8-12	2-3	45s
CORE					
Abs	Basic Leg Lift	pg. 221	8-12	2-3	45s
Lower	Basic V-twists	pg. 227	8-12	2-3	45s
Upper	Basic Crunch	pg. 215	8-12	2-3	45s
Lower Back	Intermediate Superman	pg. 210	8-12	2-3	45s

Flexibility:

Muscle	Stretch		Hold	Sets
LOWER BODY				
Quad	Standing Quads Stretch	pg. 235	30-60s	1
Hamstring	Hamstring Stretch	pg. 235	30-60s	1
Glutes	Tree Glute Stretch	pg. 236	30-60s	1
Calves	Toes Up Stretch	pg. 235	30-60s	1
Thighs	Feet First Stretch	pg. 237	30-60s	1

For those who have started the program with P1 and have worked through P2, this is now the point when you and others are noticing and commenting on your transformation. Use these positive results as the Power to keep going.

BRONZE
Program 3

During the last month of your transformation, try circuit training. This is where there's a cardio session between each strength training exercise. It gets your heart rate up and burns fat fast!

Circuit Training: Circuit training develops strength, flexibility, cardiovascular health, coordination and endurance at the same time. It consists of a wide variety of short exercises in one session, with a minimal amount of rest.

These are two tough programs. You will most definitely need determination! You have conditioned your body now to the point where you can ramp it up to new/ higher levels.

Schedule
Bronze Program 3

	Monday	Tuesday	Wednesday	Thursday	Friday	Saturday	Sunday
Week 9	**Strength:** *Upper Body* *reps: 10 sets: 2* *Circuit:* **Flexibility:**	**Cardio** *Walk:* *30-35 mins* **Flexibility:**	**Strength:** *Lower Body* *reps: 10 sets: 2* *Circuit:* **Flexibility:**	**Cardio** *Walk:* *30-35 mins* **Flexibility:**	**Strength:** *Upper Body* *reps: 10 sets: 2* *Circuit:* **Flexibility:**	**Cardio** *Walk:* *30-35 mins* **Flexibility:**	**Rest**
Week 10	**Strength:** *Lower Body* *reps: 12 sets: 2* *Circuit:* **Flexibility:**	**Cardio** *Walk:* *30-35 mins* **Flexibility:**	**Strength:** *Upper Body* *reps: 12 sets: 2* *Circuit:* **Flexibility:**	**Cardio** *Walk:* *30-35 mins* **Flexibility:**	**Strength:** *Lower Body* *reps: 12 sets: 2* *Circuit:* **Flexibility:**	**Cardio** *Walk:* *30-35 mins* **Flexibility:**	**Rest**
Week 11	**Strength:** *Upper Body* *reps: 10 sets: 3* *Circuit:* **Flexibility:**	**Cardio** *Walk:* *30-35 mins* **Flexibility:**	**Strength:** *Lower Body* *reps: 10 sets: 3* *Circuit:* **Flexibility:**	**Cardio** *Walk:* *30-35 mins* **Flexibility:**	**Strength:** *Upper Body* *reps: 10 sets: 3* *Circuit:* **Flexibility:**	**Cardio** *Walk:* *30-35 mins* **Flexibility:**	**Rest**
Week 12	**Strength:** *Lower Body* *reps: 12 sets: 3* *Circuit:* **Flexibility:**	**Cardio** *Walk:* *30-35 mins* **Flexibility:**	**Strength:** *Upper Body* *reps: 12 sets: 3* *Circuit:* **Flexibility:**	**Cardio** *Walk:* *30-35 mins* **Flexibility:**	**Strength:** *Lower Body* *reps: 12 sets: 3* *Circuit:* **Flexibility:**	**Cardio** *Walk:* *30-35 mins* **Flexibility:**	**Rest**

Cardio: *"The Walk"* On cardio days, ensure you are at your target! If you are used to walking, try incorporating a few step-ups (pg. 176) or flights of stairs to increase your heart rate.

Target Heart Rate: 64% - 75%

Strength Training: *"The Stairs" "The Uphill Killer"* is pretty much just that, you complete a set of strength training followed by a flight or two of stairs. This one is completed in your home. "The Uphill Killer" is designed to be completed outside near a hill. Perform one to three flights of stairs or walking or running the hill after each set of strength training. Of course the size of the hill will determine the intensity!

- Week 9 (Reps: 10, Sets: 2)
- Week 10 (Reps: 12, Sets: 2)
- Week 11 (Reps: 10, Sets: 3)
- Week 12 (Reps: 12, Sets: 3)

Target Heart Rate: 55% - 75%

Flexibility: Gently stretch the muscles worked and any muscles that feel tight. Tune into your body and stretch accordingly. Remember to breathe deep from your diaphragm and hold each stretch for 30 - 60 seconds.

Workout

Bronze Program 3

'The Stairs' (upper body)

Cardio/Warm-up:

Muscle	Exercise
Warm-up	5 - 10 minutes HR Target 55%
Cardio	Walking/Hills/Stairs: See program HR targets and durations
Circuit	Perform 1-3 flights of stairs after each set of strength training

Strength:

Muscle	Exercise		Reps	Sets	Rest
UPPER BODY					
Chest	Lying Down Chest Press	pg. 193	8-12	2-3	30-90s
Back	Leaning Row	pg. 196	8-12	2-3	30-90s
Biceps	Hammer Curl	pg. 207	8-12	2-3	30-90s
Triceps	Bent Leg Tricep Dip	pg. 204	8-12	2-3	30-90s
Shoulders	Standing Earth Raises	pg. 201	8-12	2-3	30-90s
CORE					
Abs	Basic Sit-up	pg. 212	8-12	2-3	30-90s
Lower	Plank From Knees	pg. 218	8-12	2-3	30-90s
Obliques	Knee Side Plank	pg. 224	8-12	2-3	30-90s

Flexibility:

Muscle	Stretch		Hold	Sets
UPPER BODY				
Chest	Tree Chest Stretch	pg. 238	30-60s	1
Biceps	Thumbs Down Stretch	pg. 239	30-60s	1
Triceps	Overhead Triceps Stretch	pg. 239	30-60s	1
Shoulders	Shoulder Cross Stretch	pg. 239	30-60s	1
CORE				
Lower Back	Twist Glute Stretch	pg. 238	30-60s	1

Workout
Bronze Program 3
'The Uphill Killer' (lower body)

Cardio/Warm-up:

Muscle	Exercise
Warm-up	5 - 10 minutes HR Target 55%
Cardio	Walking/Hills/Stairs: See program HR targets and durations
Circuit	Walk/run up 1 hill after each set

Strength:

Muscle	Exercise		Reps	Sets	Rest
LOWER BODY					
Quad	Walking Lunge	pg. 171	8-12	2-3	30-90s
Hamstring	Sumo Squats	pg. 174	8-12	2-3	30-90s
Glutes	Elevated Bridges	pg. 183	8-12	2-3	30-90s
Calves	Angled Calf Raises	pg. 187	8-12	2-3	30-90s
CORE					
Abs	Lying-down Leg Lift	pg. 222	8-12	2-3	30-90s
Lower	Strong Core Crunch	pg. 216	8-12	2-3	30-90s
Lower Back	Intermediate Superman	pg. 210	8-12	2-3	30-90s

Flexibility:

Muscle	Stretch		Hold	Sets
LOWER BODY				
Quad	Standing Quads Stretch	pg. 235	30-60s	1
Hamstring	Hamstring Stretch	pg. 235	30-60s	1
Glutes	Tree Glute Stretch	pg. 236	30-60s	1
Calves	Toes Up Stretch	pg. 235	30-60s	1
Thighs	Feet First Stretch	pg. 237	30-60s	1

You have worked hard over the last 12 weeks. Your mind, body and spirit deserve some time to celebrate, recharge and refocus. Take the next week off and celebrate the progress you've made. Find your REAL Motivation and your inspiration for the next leg of your journey. Don't forget to complete your measurements and Fitness Gauge!

SILVER
Program 1

Here in the Silver level we are going to continue to build strength and endurance.

Schedule
Silver Program 1

	Monday	Tuesday	Wednesday	Thursday	Friday	Saturday	Sunday
Week 1	**Strength:** *High Base* *reps: 10 sets: 2* **Flexibility:**	**Cardio** *Run:* *30-35 mins* *3:1 (walk:run)* **Flexibility:**	**Strength:** *Low Base* *reps: 10 sets: 2* **Flexibility:**	**Cardio** *Run:* *30-35 mins* *3:1 (walk:run)* **Flexibility:**	**Strength:** *High Base* *reps: 10 sets: 2* **Flexibility:**	**Cardio** *Run:* *30-35 mins* *3:1 (walk:run)* **Flexibility:**	**Rest**
Week 2	**Strength:** *Low Base* *reps: 12 sets: 2* **Flexibility:**	**Cardio** *Run:* *30-35 mins* *2:1 (walk:run)* **Flexibility:**	**Strength:** *High Base* *reps: 12 sets: 2* **Flexibility:**	**Cardio** *Run:* *30-35 mins* *2:1 (walk:run)* **Flexibility:**	**Strength:** *Low Base* *reps: 12 sets: 2* **Flexibility:**	**Cardio** *Run:* *30-35 mins* *2:1 (walk:run)* **Flexibility:**	**Rest**

Week 3	Strength: *High Base* reps: 10 sets: 3	Cardio *Run:* *30-35 mins* *1:1 (walk:run)*	Strength: *Low Base* reps: 10 sets: 3	Cardio *Run:* *30-35 mins* *1:1 (walk:run)*	Strength: *High Base* reps: 10 sets: 3	Cardio *Run:* *30-35 mins* *1:1 (walk:run)*	Rest
	Flexibility:	Flexibility:	Flexibility:	Flexibility:	Flexibility:	Flexibility:	
Week 4	Strength: *Low Base* reps: 12 sets: 3	Cardio *Run:* *30-35 mins* *1:2 (walk:run)*	Strength: *High Base* reps: 12 sets: 3	Cardio *Run:* *30-35 mins* *1:2 (walk:run)*	Strength: *Low Base* reps: 12 sets: 3	Cardio *Run:* *30-35 mins* *1:2 (walk:run)*	Rest
	Flexibility:	Flexibility:	Flexibility:	Flexibility:	Flexibility:	Flexibility:	

Strength Training: *"The Low Base" "The High Base"* Start with a split program by alternating your upper and lower body workouts. Both "The Low Base Strength" and "The High Base Strength" are designed to be completed in your basement, however you can always take them outside to change it up to a traveling workout. A traveling workout means taking your exercises outside, performing each exercise at a certain point like either end of a block.

Target Heart Rate: 55% - 65%

Cardio: *"The Run"* In the silver program, your cardio goal is to run 30 minutes or 5 km. You might not think you're a runner but believe me, I thought that too! It does get easier. Bring some music along and lose yourself in the music (just make sure you can still hear the world around you)! Be sure to watch your form to avoid injury.

Target Heart Rate: 65% - 80%

Here is an easy way to work your way into being able to jog for a 30 - minute period. To begin, alternate between walking with running. For example, a fast walk for three minutes and a light jog for one minute.

- Week 1 - 3 min:1 min (walk:run)
- Week 2 - 2 min:1 min (walk:run)
- Week 3 - 1 min:1 min (walk:run)
- Week 4 - 1 min:2 min (walk:run)

Remember to maintain good posture while running:

- Chest high
- Shoulders back
- Eyes forward
- Light impact when you hit the ground – heel-toe action.
- Core activated
- Lead with your hips
- Breathing should be controlled: inhale for three to five steps, exhale for three to five steps

Flexibility: Gently stretch the muscles worked and any muscles that feel tight. Tune into your body and stretch accordingly. Remember to breathe deep from your diaphragm and hold each stretch for 30 - 60 seconds.

Workout
Silver Program 1
'The High Base' (upper body)

Cardio/Warm-up:

Muscle	Exercise
Warm-up	5 - 10 minutes HR Target 55%
Cardio	The Run (check program for duration)

Strength:

Muscle	Exercise		Reps	Sets	Rest
UPPER BODY					
Chest	Push-ups	pg. 189	10-12	2-3	30-60s
Back	Bent Over Row	pg. 195	10-12	2-3	30-60s
Back	Half Wall Angel	pg. 198	10-12	2-3	30-60s
Biceps	Hammer Curls	pg. 207	10-12	2-3	30-60s
Triceps	Bent Leg Tricep Dips	pg. 204	10-12	2-3	30-60s
Shoulders	Standing Earth Raises	pg. 201	10-12	2-3	30-60s
CORE					
Abs	Straight Arm Plank	pg. 219	10-12	2-3	30-60s
Lower	Lying Down Leg Lifts	pg. 222	10-12	2-3	30-60s
Lower Back	Intermediate Superman	pg. 210	10-12	2-3	30-60s

Flexibility:

Muscle	Stretch		Hold	Sets
UPPER BODY				
Chest	Tree Chest Stretch	pg. 238	30-60s	1
Biceps	Thumbs Down Stretch	pg. 239	30-60s	1
Triceps	Overhead Triceps Stretch	pg. 239	30-60s	1
Shoulders	Shoulder Cross Stretch	pg. 239	30-60s	1
CORE				
Lower Back	Twist Glute Stretch	pg. 238	30-60s	1

Workout
Silver Program 1
'The Low Base' (lower body)

Cardio/Warm-up:

Muscle	Exercise
Warm-up	5 - 10 minutes HR Target 55%
Cardio	Learn to Run (check program for duration)

Strength:

Muscle	Exercise		Reps	Sets	Rest
LOWER BODY					
Quad	Walking Lunges	pg. 171	10-12	2-3	30-60s
Hamstring	Step-ups (wide leg)	pg. 177	10-12	2-3	30-60s
Glutes	Sumo Squats	pg. 174	10-12	2-3	30-60s
Calves	Single Angled Calf Raises	pg. 187	10-12	2-3	30-60s
CORE					
Abs	Sit-ups	pg. 213	10-12	2-3	30-60s
Lower	Elevated Bridge	pg. 183	10-12	2-3	30-60s
Upper	Crunches	pg. 215	10-12	2-3	30-60s
Obliques	V-twists	pg. 227	10-12	2-3	30-60s

liv

Flexibility:

Muscle	Stretch		Hold	Sets
LOWER BODY				
Quad	Standing Quads Stretch	pg. 235	30-60s	1
Hamstring	Hamstring Stretch	pg. 235	30-60s	1
Glutes	Tree Glute Stretch	pg. 236	30-60s	1
Calves	Toes Up Stretch	pg. 235	30-60s	1
Thighs	Feet First Stretch	pg. 237	30-60s	1
CORE				
Lower Back	Twist Glute Stretch	pg. 238	30-60s	1

You've done it! I bet you feel proud of yourself and ready to move on to the next level. Now that you've found some of your power, use it in the next phase of your training for the Silver!

SILVER
Program 2

In weeks 5-8 you can make it into a timed circuit by performing each exercise for a certain amount of time, such as 30-75 seconds.

Schedule
Silver Program 2

	Monday	Tuesday	Wednesday	Thursday	Friday	Saturday	Sunday
Week 5	**Strength:** *Upper Body Circuit: time: 30s* Flexibility:	**Cardio:** *Run: 30-35 mins 1:3(walk:run)* Flexibility:	**Strength:** *Lower Body Circuit: time: 30s* Flexibility:	**Cardio:** *Run: 30-35 mins 1:3 (walk:run)* Flexibility:	**Strength:** *Core Circuit: time: 30s* Flexibility:	**Cardio:** *Run: 30-35 mins 1:3 (walk:run)* Flexibility:	**Rest**
Week 6	**Upper Body** *Upper Body Circuit: time: 45s* Flexibility:	**Cardio** *Run: 30-35 mins 1:4 (walk:run)* Flexibility:	**Lower Body or Rest** *Lower Body Circuit: time: 45s* Flexibility:	**Cardio** *Run: 30-35 mins 1:4 (walk:run)* Flexibility:	**Core** *Core Circuit: time: 45s* Flexibility:	**Cardio** *Run: 30-35 mins 1:4 (walk:run)* Flexibility:	**Rest**

Week 7	Strength: *Upper Body Circuit:* *time: 60s*	Cardio: *Run:* *30-35 mins* *1:5 (walk:run)*	Strength: *Lower Body Circuit:* *time: 60s*	Cardio: *Run:* *30-35 mins* *1:5 (walk:run)*	Strength: *Core Circuit:* *time: 60s*	Cardio: *Run:* *30-35 mins* *1:5 (walk:run)*	Rest
	Flexibility:	**Flexibility:**	**Flexibility:**	**Flexibility:**	**Flexibility:**	**Flexibility:**	
Week 8	Strength: *Upper Body Circuit:* *time: 75s*	Cardio: *Run:* *30-35 mins* *1:6 (walk:run)*	Strength: *Lower Body Circuit:* *time: 75s*	Cardio: *Run:* *30-35 mins* *1:6 (walk:run)*	Strength: *Core Circuit:* *time: 75s*	Cardio: *Run:* *30-35 mins* *1:6 (walk:run)*	Rest
	Flexibility:	**Flexibility:**	**Flexibility:**	**Flexibility:**	**Flexibility:**	**Flexibility:**	

Cardio: *"The Run"* For cardio, continue with training to be able to run consistently for 5 km. This time try:

- Week 5 - 1 min:3 min (walk:run)
- Week 6 - 1 min:4 min (walk:run)
- Week 7 - 1 min:5 min (walk:run)
- Week 8 - 1 min:6 min (walk:run)

Target Heart Rate: 55% - 70%

Strength Training: *"The Up Time" "The Core Time" and "The Down Time"* are programs where you alternate strength and cardio exercises for a certain amount of time. The time and the number of rounds will be determined by where you are at the moment. Increase the time of each exercise or the number of rounds that you perform. This one is also great to do with your spouse or family member! *(You will require a stop-watch to time you rounds)*

Week 1: 30 sec Rounds, 2-3
Week 2: 45 sec Rounds, 2-3
Week 3: 60 sec Rounds, 2-4
Week 4: 75 sec Rounds, 2-4
* Rest 1-2 minutes after completing each round

If you are finding it to hard to complete this program, remove a cardio day and use it as a rest day instead. Remember, quality over quantity!

Target Heart Rate: 55% - 80%

Flexibility: Gently stretch the muscles worked and any muscles that feel tight. Tune into your body and stretch accordingly. Remember to breathe deep from your diaphragm and hold each stretch for 30 - 60 seconds.

liv

Workout

Silver Program 2

'The Up Time' (upper body)

Cardio/Warm-up:

Muscle	Exercise
Warm-up	5 - 10 minutes HR Target 55%
Cardio	Learn to Run (check program for duration)
Circuit	Mountain Climbers, Jumping Jacks, High Knees, Bum Kicks, Shuffles

Strength:

Muscle	Exercise		Duration	Rest
UPPER BODY				
Chest	Push-ups	pg. 189	30-75s	60-120s
Back	Bent Over Row	pg. 195	30-75s	60-120s
Biceps	Hammer Curls	pg. 207	30-75s	60-120s
Triceps	Bent Leg Tricep Dip	pg. 204	30-75s	60-120s
Shoulders	Standing Earth Raises	pg. 201	30-75s	60-120s

Flexibility:

Muscle	Stretch		Hold	Sets
UPPER BODY				
Chest	Tree Chest Stretch	pg. 238	30-60s	1
Biceps	Thumbs Down Stretch	pg. 239	30-60s	1
Triceps	Overhead Triceps Stretch	pg. 239	30-60s	1
Shoulders	Shoulder Cross Stretch	pg. 239	30-60s	1
CORE				
Lower Back	Twist Glute Stretch	pg. 238	30-60s	1

Workout
Silver Program 2
'The Down Time' (lower body)

Cardio/Warm-up:

Muscle	Exercise
Warm-up	5 - 10 minutes HR Target 55%
Cardio	Learn to Run (check program for duration)
Circuit	Mountain Climbers, Jumping Jacks, High Knees, Bum Kicks, Shuffles

Strength:

Muscle	Exercise		Duration	Rest
LOWER BODY				
Quad	Walking Lunges	pg. 171	30-75s	60-120s
Hamstring	Step-ups (wide leg)	pg. 177	30-75s	60-120s
Glutes	Reverse One Legged Dips	pg. 179	30-75s	60-120s
Calves	Angled Calf Raises	pg. 187	30-75s	60-120s

Flexibility:

Muscle	Stretch		Hold	Sets
LOWER BODY				
Quad	Leaning Quad Stretch	pg. 236	30-60s	1
Hamstring	One Seated Hamstring Stretch	pg. 236	30-60s	1
Glutes	Leg Back Glute Stretch	pg. 237	30-60s	1
Calves	Toes Up Stretch	pg. 235	30-60s	1
Thighs	Feet First Stretch	pg. 237	30-60s	1
CORE				
Lower Back	Twist Glute Stretch	pg. 238	30-60s	1

liv

Workout
Silver Program 2
'The Core Time'

Cardio/Warm-up:

Muscle	Exercise
Warm-up	5 - 10 minutes HR Target 55%
Cardio	Learn to Run (check program for duration)
Circuit	Mountain Climbers, Jumping Jacks, High Knees, Bum Kicks, Shuffles

Strength:

Muscle	Exercise		Duration	Rest
CORE				
Abs	Basic Sit-ups	pg. 212	30s - 75s	60-120s
Lower	Elevated Bridge	pg. 183	30s - 75s	60-120s
Upper	Strong Core Crunch	pg. 216	30s - 75s	60-120s
Obliques	Toe Side Plank	pg. 225	30s - 75s	60-120s
Lower Back	Flying Superman	pg. 211	30s - 75s	60-120s

Flexibility:

Muscle	Stretch		Hold	Sets
LOWER BODY				
Quad	Leaning Quad Stretch	pg. 236	30-60s	1
Hamstring	One Seated Hamstring Stretch	pg. 236	30-60s	1
Glutes	Leg Back Glute Stretch	pg. 237	30-60s	1
Calves	Toes Up Stretch	pg. 235	30-60s	1
Thighs	Feet First Stretch	pg. 237	30-60s	1
CORE				
Lower Back	Twist Glute Stretch	pg. 238	30-60s	1

After this, seeing your results in the mirror will be like Christmas. Revel in the results, this is an incredible achievement. Enjoy this realization.

SILVER
Program 3

For your last workout, try something that combines the two, design your work outs based on goals. If weight loss is your goal, then do more circuit training. If you want to gain more definition, perform your strength training exercises as supersets. You have enough knowledge now to know what you want and how to get it!

Schedule
Silver Program 3

	Monday	Tuesday	Wednesday	Thursday	Friday	Saturday	Sunday
Week 9	**Strength:** *Upper Body Super Sets: reps: 10 sets: 2* **Flexibility:**	**Cardio** *Run: 30-35 mins 1:8 (walk:run)* **Flexibility:**	**Strength:** *Lower Body Super Sets: reps: 10 sets 2* **Flexibility:**	**Cardio** *Run: 30-35 mins 1:8 (walk:run)* **Flexibility:**	**Strength:** *Upper Body Super Sets: reps: 10 sets 2* **Flexibility:**	**Cardio** *Run: 30-35 mins 1:8 (walk:run)* **Flexibility:**	**Rest**
Week 10	**Strength:** *Lower Body Super Sets: reps: 12 sets: 2* **Flexibility:**	**Cardio** *Run: 30-35 mins 1:10 (walk:run)* **Flexibility:**	**Strength:** *Upper Body Super Sets: reps: 12 sets: 2* **Flexibility:**	**Cardio** *Run: 30-35 mins 1:10 (walk:run)* **Flexibility:**	**Strength:** *Lower Body SuperSets: reps: 12 sets: 2* **Flexibility:**	**Cardio** *Run: 30-35 mins 1:10 (walk:run)* **Flexibility:**	**Rest**
Week 11	**Strength:** *Upper Body Super Sets: reps: 10 sets: 3* **Flexibility:**	**Cardio** *Run: 30-35 mins 1:15 (walk:run)* **Flexibility:**	**Strength:** *Lower Body Super Sets: reps: 10 sets: 3* **Flexibility:**	**Cardio** *Run: 30-35 mins 1:15 (walk:run)* **Flexibility:**	**Strength:** *Upper Body Super Sets: reps: 10 sets: 3* **Flexibility:**	**Cardio** *Run: 30-35 mins 1:15 (walk:run)* **Flexibility:**	**Rest**
Week 10	**Strength:** *Lower Body Super Sets: reps: 12 sets: 3* **Flexibility:**	**Cardio** *Run: 30-35 mins 1:30 (walk:run)* **Flexibility:**	**Strength:** *Upper Body Super Sets: reps: 12 sets: 3* **Flexibility:**	**Cardio** *Run: 30-35 mins 1:30 (walk:run)* **Flexibility:**	**Strength:** *Lower Body Super Sets: reps: 12 sets: 3* **Flexibility:**	**Cardio** *Run: 30-35 mins 1:30 (walk:run)* **Flexibility:**	**Rest**

liv

Cardio: *"The Run"* For your cardio you are in the home stretch to run 5 km. Don't give up. Continue increasing your endurance to the finish line.

- Week 9 - 1 min:8 min (walk:run)
- Week 10 - 1 min:10 min (walk:run)
- Week 11 - 1 min:15 min (walk:run)
- Week 12 - 1 min:30 min (walk:run)

Target Heart Rate: 55% - 70%

Strength Training: *"Super Sets"* For your last workout you might want to try Super Setting. You will gain more definition, become stronger and increase your inner strength.

Target Heart Rate: 50% - 70%

Super-sets: Super sets are when you do two exercises for a particular muscle or muscle groups sequentially. For example, try doing a set of lunges followed by a set of squats, or a chest press followed by push-ups. It's going to be tough. This is where you will have to dig deep, use your REAL Motivation, affirmations and power words. Get into your soundtrack and get ready!

Continue to push yourself to new heights. You now have the strength and power of mind and body to bring home the silver.

Flexibility: Gently stretch the muscles worked and any muscles that feel tight. Tune into your body and stretch accordingly. Remember to breathe deep from your diaphragm and hold each stretch for 30 - 60 seconds.

Workouts
Silver Program 3
'The High Super Set' (upper body)

Cardio/Warm-up:

Muscle	Exercise
Warm-up	5 - 10 minutes HR Target 55%
Cardio	Learn to Run (check program for duration)

Strength:

Muscle	Exercise		Reps	Sets	Rest
UPPER BODY					
Chest	Push-ups Lying Down Chest Press	pg. 189 pg. 193	10-12 each	2-3	60s
Back	Bent Over Row The Full Angels	pg. 195 pg. 199	10-12 each	2-3	60s
Biceps	Twenty Ones Hammer Curl	pg. 208 pg. 207	10-12 each	2-3	60s
Triceps	Bent Leg Tricep Dips Standing Tricep Extensions	pg. 204 pg. 203	10-12 each	2-3	60s
Shoulders	Standing Earth Raises Front & Side Earth Raisers	pg. 201 pg. 202	10-12 each	2-3	60s
CORE					
Abs	Sit-ups	pg. 213	10-12	2-3	60s
Lower	Lying-down Leg Lift	pg. 222	10-12	2-3	60s
Obliques	Weighted V-twist	pg. 228	10-12	2-3	60s
Lower Back	Flying Superman	pg. 211	10-12	2-3	60s

Flexibility:

Muscle	Stretch		Hold	Sets
UPPER BODY				
Chest	Tree Chest Stretch	pg. 238	30-60s	1
Biceps	Thumbs Down Stretch	pg. 239	30-60s	1
Triceps	Overhead Triceps Stretch	pg. 239	30-60s	1
Shoulders	Shoulder Cross Stretch	pg. 239	30-60s	1
CORE				
Lower Back	Twist Glute Stretch	pg. 238	30-60s	1

liv

Workouts
Silver Program 3
'The Low Super Set' (lower body)

Cardio/Warm-up:

Muscle	Exercise
Warm-up	5 - 10 minutes HR Target 55%
Cardio	Learn to Run (check program for duration)

Strength:

Muscle	Exercise		Reps	Sets	Rest
LOWER BODY					
Quad	Walking Lunges Step-ups (wide leg)	pg. 171 pg. 177	10-12 each	2-3	60s
Hamstring	Reverse Leg Dips Sumo Squats	pg. 180 pg. 174	10-12 each	2-3	60s
Glutes	Elevated Bridge Crunch - Straight Legged Bridge	pg. 183 pg. 184	10-12 each	2-3	60s
Calves	Single Calf Raise Angled Calf Raise	pg. 187 pg. 187	10-12 each	2-3	60s
CORE					
Abs	Straight Arm Plank	pg. 219	10-12	2-3	60s
Lower	Advanced Leg Lift	pg. 223	10-12	2-3	60s
Upper	Toes Side Plank	pg. 225	10-12	2-3	60s
Obliques	Weighted V-twist	pg. 228	10-12	2-3	60s

Flexibility:

Muscle	Stretch		Hold	Sets
LOWER BODY				
Quad	Standing Quads Stretch	pg. 235	30-60s	1
Hamstring	Hamstring Stretch	pg. 235	30-60s	1
Glutes	Tree Glute Stretch	pg. 236	30-60s	1
Calves	Toes Up Stretch	pg. 235	30-60s	1
Thighs	Feet First Stretch	pg. 237	30-60s	1
CORE				
Lower Back	Twist Glute Stretch	pg. 238	30-60s	1

Stand back and look at how fearless you have become! The strength and wisdom that you have gained from this journey is an inspiration to yourself, as well as the people around you. You now have the power to go for the Gold!

You have worked hard over the last 13 weeks. Your mind, body and spirit deserve some time to rest, recharge and refocus. Take the next week off and reflect on the progress you've made. Use your REAL Motivation card to find inspiration for the next leg of your journey.

GOLD
Program 1

This is where you take everything that you've learned and go to the next level. You've built your foundation, you've increased your cardiovascular strength and you're kinesthetically aware of your posture and movements.

Schedule
Gold Program 1

	Monday	Tuesday	Wednesday	Thursday	Friday	Saturday	Sunday
Week 1	**Strength:** *Upper Body* *reps: 50* **Flexibility:**	**Cardio** *Active Recovery:* *30-35 mins* **Flexibility:**	**Strength:** *Lower Body* *reps: 50* **Flexibility:**	**Cardio** *Active Recovery:* *30-35 mins* **Flexibility:**	**Strength:** *Upper Body* *reps: 50* **Flexibility:**	**Cardio** *Active Recovery:* *30-35 mins* **Flexibility:**	**Rest**
Week 2	**Strength:** *Lower Body* *reps: 50* **Flexibility:**	**Cardio** *Active Recovery:* *30-35 mins* **Flexibility:**	**Strength:** *Upper Body* *reps: 50* **Flexibility:**	**Cardio** *Run:* *30-35 mins* **Flexibility:**	**Strength:** *Lower Body* *reps: 50* **Flexibility:**	**Cardio** *Active Recovery:* *30-35 mins* **Flexibility:**	**Rest**
Week 3	**Strength:** *Upper Body* *reps: 50* **Flexibility:**	**Cardio** *Active Recovery:* *30-35 mins* **Flexibility:**	**Strength:** *Lower Body* *reps: 50* **Flexibility:**	**Cardio** *Active Recovery:* *30-35 mins* **Flexibility:**	**Strength:** *Upper Body* *reps: 50* **Flexibility:**	**Cardio** *Active Recovery:* *30-35 mins* **Flexibility:**	**Rest**

liv

Week 4	Strength: Lower Body reps: 50	Cardio Active Recovery: 30-35 mins	Strength: Upper Body reps: 50	Cardio Active Recovery: 30-35 mins	Strength: Lower Body reps: 50	Cardio Active Recovery: 30-35 mins	Rest
	Flexibility:	Flexibility:	Flexibility:	Flexibility:	Flexibility:	Flexibility:	

Cardio: *"The Easy"* I suggest that you use your cardio days as an active recovery. This means a light jog, a brisk walk or a nice bike ride. Enjoy this time and allow your mind and body to heal from such intensity!

Target Heart Rate: 55% - 65%

Strength Training: *"The 50s"* The 50s strength training is a tough one. I suggest that you use your cardio days as an active recovery. This means a light jog, a brisk walk or a nice bike ride. Enjoy this time and allow your mind and body to heal from the intensity of the 50s.

Target Heart Rate: 60% - 90%

*If you're finding it too difficult, scale down the repetitions from 50 to 40 or 30. You might also want to give yourself a few workout passes. 1 pass = 5 walking steps For example: If you use one pass you world perform 45 reps followed by 5 walking steps; use 2 passes and do 40 reps and 10 walking steps.

Flexibility: Gently stretch the muscles worked and any muscles that feel tight. Tune into your body and stretch accordingly. Remember to breathe deep from your diaphragm and hold each stretch for 30 - 60 seconds.

Workouts
Gold Program 1
'The High 50s' (upper body)

Cardio/Warm-up:

Muscle	Exercise
Warm-up	5 - 10 minutes HR Target 55%
The Easy	Light Jog, Brisk Walk, Bike Ride
50s	Mountain Climbers, Side Walk Kicks, Bum Kicks, Grape Vine, Step-ups, High Knees

Strength:

Muscle	Exercise		Reps	Sets	Rest
UPPER BODY					
Chest	Push-ups	pg. 189	50	1	60-90s
Back	Full Wall Angels	pg. 199	50	1	60-90s
Biceps	Hammer Curls	pg. 207	50	1	60-90s
Triceps	Straight Leg Tricep Dips	pg. 205	50	1	60-90s
Shoulders	Front & Side Earth Raisers	pg. 202	50	1	60-90s
CORE					
Abs	Sit-ups	pg. 213	50	1	60-90s
Lower	Lying-down Leg Lift	pg. 222	50	1	60-90s
Obliques	Weighted V-twist	pg. 228	50	1	60-90s
Lower Back	Flying Superman	pg. 211	50	1	60-90s

Flexibility:

Muscle	Stretch		Hold	Sets
UPPER BODY				
Chest	Tree Chest Stretch	pg. 238	30-60s	1
Biceps	Thumbs Down Stretch	pg. 239	30-60s	1
Triceps	Overhead Triceps Stretch	pg. 239	30-60s	1
Shoulders	Shoulder Cross Stretch	pg. 239	30-60s	1
CORE				
Lower Back	Twist Glute Stretch	pg. 238	30-60s	1

Workouts

Gold Program 1

'The Low 50s' (lower body)

Cardio/Warm-up:

Muscle	Exercise
Warm-up	5 - 10 minutes HR Target 55%
The Easy	Light Jog, Brisk Walk, Bike Ride
50s	Mountain Climbers, Side Walk Kicks, Bum Kicks, Grape Vine, Step-ups

Strength:

Muscle	Exercise		Reps	Sets	Rest
LOWER BODY					
Quad	Uphill Lunges	pg. 172	50	1	60-90s
Hamstring	Jumping Squats	pg. 175	50	1	60-90s
Glutes	Straight Legged Bridge	pg. 184	50	1	60-90s
Calves	Single Calf Raise	pg. 186	50	1	60-90s
CORE					
Abs	Advanced Sit-up Crunches	pg. 214 pg. 215	50 50	1 1	60-90s 60-90s
Obliques	Leaned Back V-twist	pg. 229	50	1	60-90s

Flexibility:

Muscle	Stretch		Hold	Sets
LOWER BODY				
Quad	Standing Quads Stretch	pg. 235	30-60s	1
Hamstring	Hamstring Stretch	pg. 235	30-60s	1
Glutes	Leg Back Glute Stretch	pg. 237	30-60s	1
Calves	Toes Up Stretch	pg. 235	30-60s	1
Thighs	Feet First Stretch	pg. 237	30-60s	1
CORE				
Lower Back	Twist Glute Stretch	pg. 238	30-60s	1

GOLD
Program 2

Next step? Push harder in Gold P2. Be proud of your determination. Be ready to dig even deeper to get your inner fire burning. These workouts are amazing not only for your body, but your mind and your spirit as well!

Schedule
Gold Program 2

	Monday	Tuesday	Wednesday	Thursday	Friday	Saturday	Sunday
Week 5	**Strength:** *Full Body* *reps: 10 sets: 2*	**Cardio** *Interval:* *30-35 mins*	**Strength:** *Full Body* *reps: 10 sets: 2*	**Cardio** *Active Recovery* *Light Jog* *30-35 mins*	**Strength:** *Full Body* *reps: 10 sets: 2*	**Cardio** *Interval:* *30-35 mins*	**Rest**
	Flexibility:	**Flexibility:**	**Flexibility:**	**Flexibility:**	**Flexibility:**	**Flexibility:**	
Week 6	**Strength:** *Full Body* *reps: 12 sets: 2*	**Cardio** *Interval:* *30-35 mins*	**Strength:** *Full Body* *reps: 12 sets: 2*	**Cardio** *Active Recovery* *Light Jog* *30-35 mins*	**Strength:** *Full Body* *reps: 12 sets: 2*	**Cardio** *Interval:* *30-35 mins*	**Rest**
	Flexibility:	**Flexibility:**	**Flexibility:**	**Flexibility:**	**Flexibility:**	**Flexibility:**	
Week 7	**Strength:** *Full Body* *reps: 10 sets: 3*	**Cardio** *Interval:* *30-35 mins*	**Strength:** *Full Body* *reps: 10 sets: 3*	**Cardio** *Active Recovery* *Light Jog* *30-35 mins*	**Strength:** *Full Body* *reps: 10 sets: 3*	**Cardio** *Interval:* *30-35 mins*	**Rest**
	Flexibility:	**Flexibility:**	**Flexibility:**	**Flexibility:**	**Flexibility:**	**Flexibility:**	
Week 8	**Strength:** *Full Body* *reps: 12 sets: 3*	**Cardio** *Interval:* *30-35 mins*	**Strength:** *Full Body* *reps: 12 sets: 3*	**Cardio** *Active Recovery* *Light Jog* *30-35 mins*	**Strength:** *Full Body* *reps: 12 sets: 3*	**Cardio** *Interval:* *30-35 mins*	**Rest**
	Flexibility:	**Flexibility:**	**Flexibility:**	**Flexibility:**	**Flexibility:**	**Flexibility:**	

liv

Aerobic: Means "with oxygen." Improves your cardiovascular system's efficiency while absorbing and transporting oxygen. Jogging and swimming are examples of aerobic exercise.

Anaerobic: Means "without oxygen." Builds strength, power and muscle mass. Anaerobic systems come in either anaerobic glycolysis or ATP-CP forms. Weightlifting and jumping rope are examples of anaerobic exercise.

Anaerobic Glycolysis: The first anaerobic system. It doesn't require oxygen, but does use lactic acid in actions lasting longer than a few seconds. Sprinting is an example of an exercise that uses anaerobic glycolysis.

ATP-CP: ATP, also known as adenosine triphosphate, is your body's energy currency, used to perform any activity. CP stands for creatine phosphate. ATP-CP is the second anaerobic system. It's found in muscle fibres and doesn't use or produce any oxygen. It's used for quick actions of the body, like spiking in volleyball.

Cardio: *"The Killer"* is the cardio component of this program. It's called "The Killer" because you're increasing your intensity as you activate different energy systems. (see side panel) It requires you to have your mind open to allow your spirit to come through.

Target Heart Rate: 70% - 95%

Warm up for 3-5 minutes. Then, increase your intensity every 50-100 steps as you move through the exercise scale (pg. 96). Repeat for the duration. For Example:

Exercise (Steps 50-100)	Intensity Level
Warm-up (3-5 mins)	5
Brisk Walk	6
Light Jog	7
Fast Jog	8
Sprint	9
Brisk Walk	6
Light Jog	7
Fast Jog	8
Sprint	9

Strength Training: *"The Power"* In this program, the strength training exercises are a full body exercise, or a combination of a lower and upper body to make a full body component. What's great with these exercises is you get the best bang for your buck.

Target Heart Rate: 60% - 80%

Flexibility: Gently stretch the muscles worked and any muscles that feel tight. Tune into your body and stretch accordingly. Remember to breathe deep from your diaphragm and hold each stretch for 30 - 60 seconds.

Workouts
Gold Program 2
'The Power'

Cardio/Warm-up:

Muscle	Exercise
Warm-up	5 -10 minutes HR Target 55%
Cardio	Intervals (check interval description)

Strength:

Muscle	Exercise		Reps	Sets	Rest
FULL BODY					
Quad / Shoulders	Uphill Lunges Earth Raisers	pg. 172 pg. 201	12-15	3-5	30s-60s
Hamstring / Triceps	Touch Squats Tricep Dips	pg. 173 pg. 205	12-15	3-5	30s-60s
Glutes / Biceps	Wide Leg Set-up Hammer Curl	pg. 177 pg. 207	12-15	3-5	30s-60s
Full Body	Burpies Push-ups	pg. 233 pg. 190	12-15	3-5	30s-60s
CORE					
Core / Back	Walking Inch Worm Single Arm Row	pg. 220 pg. 194	12-15	3-5	30s-60s
Obliques	Twist Side Plank	pg. 236	12-15	3-5	30s-60s

Flexibility:

Muscle	Stretch		Hold	Sets
LOWER BODY				
Quad	Leaning Quad Stretch	pg. 236	30-60s	1
Hamstring	One Seated Hamstring Stretch	pg. 236	30-60s	1
Glutes	Leg Back Glute Stretch	pg. 237	30-60s	1
Calves	Toes Up Stretch	pg. 235	30-60s	1
Thighs	Feet First Stretch	pg. 237	30-60s	1
UPPER BODY				
Chest	Tree Chest Stretch	pg. 238	30-60s	1
Biceps	Thumbs Down Stretch	pg. 239	30-60s	1
Triceps	Overhead Triceps Stretch	pg. 239	30-60s	1
Shoulders	Shoulder Cross Stretch	pg. 239	30-60s	1
CORE				
Lower Back	Twist Glute Stretch	pg. 238	30-60s	1

GOLD
Program 3

Congratulations – you've almost made it to the finish line. Keep your head up; there are just a couple more workouts left to go!

Schedule
Gold Program 3

	Monday	Tuesday	Wednesday	Thursday	Friday	Saturday	Sunday
Week 9	**Strength:** *Full Body reps: 12,10,8,10,12 sets: 5* **Flexibility:**	**Cardio** *30-35 mins* **Flexibility:**	**Strength:** *Full Body reps: 12,10,8,10,12 sets: 5* **Flexibility:**	**Cardio** *30-35 mins* **Flexibility:**	**Strength:** *Full Body reps: 12,10,8,10,12 sets: 5* **Flexibility:**	**Cardio** *30-35 mins* **Flexibility:**	**Rest**
Week 10	**Strength:** *Full Body reps: 12,10,8,10,12 sets: 5* **Flexibility:**	**Cardio** *30-35 mins* **Flexibility:**	**Strength:** *Full Body reps: 12,10,8,10,12 sets: 5* **Flexibility:**	**Cardio** *30-35 mins* **Flexibility:**	**Strength:** *Full Body reps: 12,10,8,10,12 sets: 5* **Flexibility:**	**Cardio** *30-35 mins* **Flexibility:**	**Rest**
Week 11	**Strength:** *Full Body reps: 12,10,8,10,12 sets: 5* **Flexibility:**	**Cardio** *30-35 mins* **Flexibility:**	**Strength:** *Full Body reps: 12,10,8,10,12 sets: 5* **Flexibility:**	**Cardio** *30-35 mins* **Flexibility:**	**Strength:** *Full Body reps: 12,10,8,10,12 sets: 5* **Flexibility:**	**Cardio** *30-35 mins* **Flexibility:**	**Rest**
Week 12	**Strength:** *Full Body reps: 12,10,8,10,12 sets: 5* **Flexibility:**	**Cardio** *30-35 mins* **Flexibility:**	**Strength:** *Full Body reps: 12,10,8,10,12 sets: 5* **Flexibility:**	**Cardio** *30-35 mins* **Flexibility:**	**Strength:** *Full Body reps: 12,10,8,10,12 sets: 5* **Flexibility:**	**Cardio** *30-35 mins* **Flexibility:**	**Rest**

Cardio: *"The Groove"* I think by far this is my favourite cardio session. Listen to your soundtrack and perform a different cardio activity for the duration of each song. Get creative – dance, move, jump, skip or whatever you like for each song and get your heart pumping!

Target Heart Rate: 60% - 90%

Strength Training: *"Pyramid Training"* This is the last tough workout. If you've come this far, you can make it through. "Pyramid Training" is designed to keep your body guessing what's next. In this program you are going to mix it up by using pyramid training instead of the traditional number of sets. Do 5 sets with the following reps: 12, 10, 8, 10, 12.

Target Heart Rate: 60% - 80%

Flexibility: Gently stretch the muscles worked and any muscles that feel tight. Tune into your body and stretch accordingly. Remember to breathe deep from your diaphragm and hold each stretch for 30 - 60 seconds.

Workouts
Gold Program 3
'The Hill'

Cardio/Warm-up:

Muscle	Exercise
Warm-up	5 - 10 minutes HR Target 55%

Strength:

Muscle	Exercise	Reps	Sets	Rest
LOWER BODY				
Quad	Lunges: walking, straight leg, angled with hands over head, walking pg. 171	12,10,8,10,12	2-3	30s-60s
Hamstring	Squats: walking sumo, walking sumo with pulse, jumping, jack meets sumo, touch pg. 174	12,10,8,10,12	2-3	30s-60s
UPPER BODY				
Chest	Push-ups: on bench, lower surface, from toes, pulse for one count, close grip pg. 189	12,10,8,10,12	2-3	30s-60s
Back	Wall Angel/Row: half wall angel, bent over row, seated row, full wall angel/forward shoulder raise, leaning row pg. 197	12,10,8,10,12	2-3	30s-60s
CORE				
Abs	Core: advanced sit-ups, advanced leg lift, twist side plank, the v-crunch, leaned back v-twist pg. 209	12,10,8,10,12	2-3	30s-60s

Flexibility:

Muscle	Stretch		Hold	Sets
LOWER BODY				
Quad	Leaning Quad Stretch	pg. 236	30-60s	1
Hamstring	One Seated Hamstring Stretch	pg. 236	30-60s	1
Glutes	Leg Back Glute Stretch	pg. 237	30-60s	1
Calves	Toes Up Stretch	pg. 235	30-60s	1
Thighs	Feet First Stretch	pg. 237	30-60s	1
UPPER BODY				
Chest	Tree Chest Stretch	pg. 238	30-60s	1
Biceps	Thumbs Down Stretch	pg. 239	30-60s	1
Triceps	Overhead Tricep Stretch	pg. 239	30-60s	1
Shoulders	Shoulder Cross Stretch	pg. 239	30-60s	1
CORE				
Lower Back	Twist Glute Stretch	pg. 238	30-60s	1

Workouts
Gold Program 3
'The Groove'

Cardio/Warm-up:

Muscle	Exercise
Warm-up	5 - 10 minutes HR Target 55%
Cardio	Perform each exercise for the duration of a song from your soundtrack: High Knees, Bum Kicks, Step-ups, Shuffles, Jumping Jacks, Stairs, Sprints, Dancing, Mountain Climbers, Skipping

You made it! You earn the Gold! Whether you began this program three, six or nine months ago, you've conditioned your body to a level of fitness that's truly inspiring.

Take some time to reflect on how far you've come. I suspect that your transformation has been more than a physical change. Perhaps you're beginning to really feel and believe in your personal power. With your renewed strength, you can create the life you desire and live your dreams. Wherever this leads you, know each step was achieved.

You have worked hard over the last 12 weeks. Your mind, body and spirit deserve some time to rest, recharge and refocus. Take the next week off and celebrate the progress you've made. Create a new REAL Motivation card to find inspiration for the next leg of your journey.

Customize your own Program

Use the blank forms below to create your own customized program.

Schedule

	Monday	Tuesday	Wednesday	Thursday	Friday	Saturday	Sunday
Week							
Week							
Week							
Week							

Cardio: _____

_____

_____

Target Heart Rate: _____

Strength: _____

_____

_____

Workouts

Cardio/Warm-up:

Muscle	Exercise
Warm-up	
Cardio	

Strength:

Muscle	Exercise	Reps	Sets	Rest
LOWER BODY				
Quad				
Hamstring				
Glutes				
Calves				
UPPER BODY				
Chest				
Back				
Biceps				
Triceps				
Shoulders				
CORE				
Abs				
Lower				
Upper				
Obliques				
Lower Back				

Flexibility:

Muscle	Exercise	Hold	Sets
LOWER BODY			
Quad			
Hamstring			
Glutes			
Calves			
UPPER BODY			
Chest			
Back			
Biceps			
Triceps			
Shoulders			
CORE			
Abs			
Lower			
Upper			
Obliques			
Lower Back			

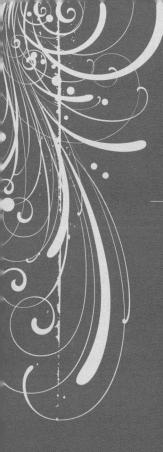

Be Truth, where there is Truth there is Expression and where there is Expression there is VOICE

Spirit

CHAPTER THIRTEEN: Healing and Nourishing Your Spirit

CHAPTER FOURTEEN: The Choice Is Yours

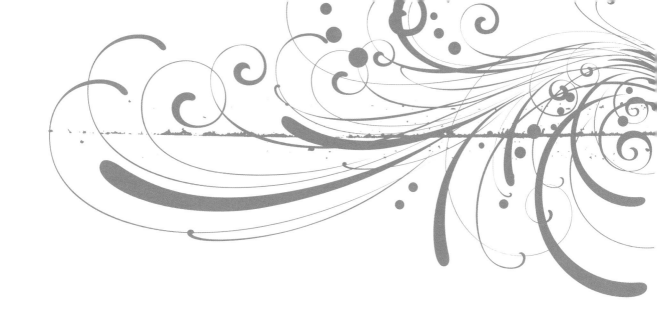

Chapter Thirteen
HEALING AND NOURISHING YOUR SPIRIT

"Love the animals, love the plants, love everything.
If you love everything, you will perceive the divine
mystery in things. Once you perceive it, you will begin to
comprehend it better every day. And you will come
at last to love the whole world
with an all-embracing love."

Fyodor Dostoyevsky

HEALING AND NOURISHING YOUR SPIRIT

Thus far, we have focused on the physical body, through hard work and perseverance we now realize it's potential. Our bodies are truly remarkable! The third aspect of the program goes beyond the mind and body to the spirit. Religious or not, you may have thought how amazing our universe is, how it sustains our billions of tiny lives revolving around space. Perhaps you have felt a connection, saw someone on a street and felt the urge to look back without knowing why. You may have felt a warm vibration or energy around you. Believing in a higher power or not, this section will deal with the energy of spirit. Read through this section and reflect on this energy and how you can use it to strengthen your life.

Healing

Trees trust in the cycle of the seasons, releasing their leaves each autumn, allowing and embracing what is to come. Freeing these leaves now creates space for new growth in the spring. We can do the same, if we trust and continue to release, we will continue to grow.

Healing is a powerful method of releasing and letting go of your mental, emotional and physical attachment to a certain situation or event. There are many powerful ways that you can heal by releasing your emotional attachments. This process can't be rushed. It all comes in perfect timing when you are ready to surrender to what that situation is trying to show you. When the dust settles you will then see the true gift that is waiting for you.

I have been through many circumstances and situations that I've had to overcome in order to see the true value of the gifts that were waiting. I was able to release all toxic energy, which allowed me to move forward finding strength, courage, endless power, peace, love and forgiveness.

148

Emotions

Many of us are filled with so much pain and hurt that we are afraid to feel and speak our true feelings. So, in order to adapt in our everyday lives, we place veils and masks over what we really feel. This is much easier than having to face and embrace the true emotions that lie deep with in all of us.

In order to truly heal, you need to feel it. You need to feel your anger, resentment, pain and hurt. We have emotions for a reason! Don't let yourself be afraid of how others will react. Expressing your emotions is critical for you to connect your body, mind and spirit. It releases stress hormones from our body. It's okay to voice your opinion, it's okay to be wrong, it's okay to make mistakes, it's okay to forgive and accept the pain that you might be feeling. I believe nothing grows without the rain, and to me, our emotional state is what allows us to conquer our dreams and grow.

Use the next 13 weeks to heal any emotional wounds that you have been carrying around. Trust me, it feels very powerful when you have released your emotional attachments to any situation.

Journaling

Journaling is an excellent way to express your thoughts, and emotions. It can be very therapeutic. There is no right or wrong way to do it. Be open. Whatever comes to mind, write it down, do not judge or evaluate, let the words flow onto the page, releasing these thoughts and feelings. It may lead you to learning, realization and freedom from emotional attachments.

I've used this method to not only journal my thoughts and emotions, but have also used it to express my voice, to heal some of my past circumstances.

There are many different methods of journaling. You may have heard of a gratitude journal or a travel journal, but try creating a "Lifestyle Journal" for this program. It doesn't have to be anything fancy - it can even be typed on your computer if you're more comfortable typing. Honestly, write out how you're feeling during this journey, the good, or, the not so good and what you have learned.

Music

Music exists in so many different forms, rap, jazz, country, hip-hop, classical and so on. Due to the diverse nature of this art, it is something most of us relate and connect to on a personal level.

Think about listening to your favorite song, or reflect on a song that you connected with during a special or challenging time in your life. This may be your wedding song, or one that reminds you of a loved one or a triumph in your life. When you hear this song, perhaps even years later you feel the emotions expressed in the lyrics, you feel the rhythm and it sparks something inside you to move freely.

I use music as a way to inspire myself to be the best that I can be. Not only with my affirmations or my visions on the REAL Motivation card, but as a means to give me the energy of spirit to know that I can truly make a difference. My theme song in life is "The River" by Garth Brooks. There is something so powerful about the lyrics in this song that it hit me right where it needs to, in my heart. It seems that this song and the lyrics spoke to me in a certain way that gave me the momentum to chase my dreams.

Your Life's Soundtrack

Create a soundtrack for your life, and include a Theme Song for Life. Your Theme Song for Life should be something that sums up your life, not so much your past, but what gives you the motivation or inspiration to keep going.

This soundtrack is going to be played while you complete your workouts. Choose eight to 15 songs that you have always loved.

This is a key component to this program so please take the time to think of songs that really mean something to you. Choose songs that make you feel energized, that bring a tear to your eye.

Track 1: _____ Track 7: _____

Track 2: _____ Track 8: _____

Track 3: _____ Track 9: _____

Track 4: _____ Track 10: _____

Track 5: _____ Track 11: _____

Track 6: _____ Track 12: _____

Theme Song for Life: _____

Nature

There is something so magical about being near nature – a flower garden, forest, the mountains, a sunset or even a flock of birds flying high. The true beauty of our planet cannot be denied. I have been blessed to experience the red mountains in Sedona, the freeness of the lakes in Ontario, the ocean in California, the lush beauty of Jamaica and Cuba, the landscapes of Arizona and Nevada and I live near the beautiful Rocky Mountains.

Through my many healing sessions, I was always drawn to nature, where I felt most comfortable surrendering my emotions. It seemed that the more time I spent in nature, either exercising, clearing my mind or having a healing session, the more I felt the energy within myself.

I have been practicing meditation in nature for years. I complete everything outside, whether it's my yoga practice by the river, or my healing sessions under my favorite tree. Just give it a try and see if you can tap into or draw on the energy of the beauty of nature that we live in.

Prayer and Meditation

We have all heard this word and I am sure many of us pray. We pray to our past loved ones, we pray to what we consider God, Source, Spirit, Buddha or Ala. We pray for health and prosperity, we pray for strength and courage and answers. If you pray, I encourage you to pray often during the next 13 weeks to strengthen your spirit and give you the power to succeed.

Meditation is a practice that quiets your mind and allows you to enter into a state of energy. Each one of us has the capacity to quiet our minds and achieve peacefulness. There are many techniques for meditating including listening to music, exercising, dancing and singing.

An easy way to begin meditating is to find a quite spot where you won't be disturbed. I recommend trying to do this after a workout. Lie or sit comfortably and focus your attention on your feet. Move your toes and then relax. Then, move to your legs. Tense your legs and then relax them. Continue this exercise of moving and relaxing as you bring your attention up your body, noticing each area and muscle, all the way to your head and face. Now, relax your body and feel it sink into the ground. Listen to the calmness of your breath as you relax your body and feel the energy that is within you. Don't force yourself to relax or worry about how long it takes. Just take slow, full breaths and focus only on your body and breathing.

Next, repeat the affirmations that help you stay focused on your journey. Continue to breathe and repeat them, as many times as you feel that is needed. Bring to mind where you are going with your REAL Motivation card. See it in your mind. See yourself owning your life in the movie that you first created. Feel your emotions as you go through it. Feel how empowered you are by taking control of your life and own every bit of it!

As you progressed you noticed that your workouts became easier as you gained strength, the same holds true with the practice of meditation. The more you work with it, the easier it becomes. Begin with short sessions and then progress into longer sessions. There is something so magical that happens when we can allow ourselves to just let go of all of our worries, our roles, our material world and focus on our spirit.

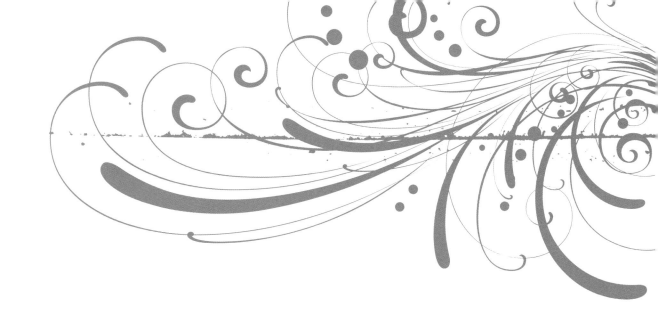

Chapter Fourteen
THE CHOICE IS YOURS

"All of the places of our lives are sanctuaries; some
of them just happen to have steeples. And all of the
people in our lives are saints; it is just that some of them
have day jobs and most will never have feast days
named for them."

Robert Benson

THE CHOICE IS YOURS

Congratulations - you have made the decision to take control of your life! It's your time to see who you can be, without limitations, creating your world as you desire it to be. Have you ever questioned why you were put on this earth, why you were given the parents, events and circumstances that are yours? Do you think that we are born into this life with no control over what we do and where we end up? Do you think that cars, homes, jobs and beauty are really just for the privileged? Do you think you are here just to fulfill the job you're in, the family role you play or even the status you hold?

Allow Your Life to be Transformed

You are reading this because you are ready for a change. But what's the real reason for this change? Is it a feeling, a way to regain control of you life or - even better - to really challenge yourself to just see how powerful you really are? You have to decide at this moment that there is no other option but to make this into an incredible change. Surrendering to it is only the beginning. The rest is allowing the true magnitude of our existence to be revealed. It is your willingness to listen and feel from your heart, which will allow your life to be transformed.

Make Decisions for the Future, Today

As you go through each day, just remember that each moment makes up our lives. It is your decision here in the present moment that makes all of this possible. Your life, your actions and your glory - it all begins here and now. Please just allow yourself to be the lead motivator in your life. There is no need to share your journey with anyone who may not be in the same space as you. You are the only one on this challenge; you are the only one you should be listening to. And above all, enjoy the journey you are about to undertake. This is about living the life you've always wanted. Let the richness of the experience sustain you.

Release the Past

Think of your house, your job, and your friends - any aspect of your life. Do you like what you see? Realize that your surroundings are only from your past thoughts and your reality for tomorrow is created today. How are we able to change the way we live if we continue to allow our lives to be repeated and evolve as they have over the last decade?

Don't beat yourself up over your past. Your vision of yourself may be filled with doubt, fear, insecurities, guilt and loss of pride. I'm here to tell you that you are so much more than those feelings. No matter what your past or actions, your opinions of yourself stand to be corrected. You are the only one in this world that has your abilities and how you discover them and use them will determine who you are. As you progress throughout the next 13 weeks, you'll begin to see your life in a different way. It is from this perspective that the real transformation occurs.

Experience Life

Too many of us allow our ego-driven minds to control our lives, thinking and believing that this is the ultimate life - the cars, the status, the larger homes and the money that we think makes the world go 'round. In order to realign yourself with your chosen path you must first enable yourself to feel the connection to the heart and spirit that is within. For starters, how do you perform your daily routine? Most of us are on autopilot and allow ourselves to be run by the same routine, same excuses day after day. We fight traffic, skip meals, complain and do nothing about it.

Take the time to find out what is truly important to you. Spend time alone envisioning your transformed life. You may find that you are being called to take a nature walk. If you're near the ocean, take your shoes off and enjoy the feeling of your toes in the sand. If you're near a creek, stand with your feet submerged. Take this time and reflect on what is meant by just living in the moment. Feel, breathe, observe. Notice any signs that come your way, whether it's a bird flying high in the sky, or a child running, or even the beauty of the sunset. Whatever it may be, just remember to be present enough to embrace the miracle, which is waiting to be received. This nourishment of the heart and spirit will allow you to find the steps on your chosen path.

Forgive

You may already know that forgiveness is the first step to changing the path of your life. Forgive those around you for the hurts they have caused. You can do this either in person or just with your thoughts. And don't forget about yourself. Forgiving self-imposed letdowns is almost more difficult than forgiving others. It takes strength, hope and faith. Forgiving and loving yourself for who you are now, is the most powerful gift you can give yourself.

Your belief system, your age and your gender don't matter; all that matters is your willingness to see and forgive all that has been in your life prior to now.

Time is an Illusion

Take away the deadlines that you have set for the achievement of your goal. Goals are good, but we can get so fixated on them and forget the journey. Remember it is one step at a time. Only one. Breathe deeply, rejuvenate your spirit and live in the moment. If you stumble, get back up and try again. Remind yourself why you are on this journey. Envision the transformed future you will enjoy, and have faith, believing in your ability to get there.

Set Intentions

If we don't act on our desires, there will be no change. Thinking about it is good, but it is action that gets you where you want to go. It doesn't matter whether you believe in a source of spirit, if that is beyond you or a greater strength within you. Trust that you can do and achieve what you want. You must be accountable to yourself to make real changes in your life. It is only when you are Real with yourself about your desires and behaviors, that true transformation will take place.

When it comes to intentions be positive, and live that positivity. Don't fall into the trap of wishing for superficial items. Yes, we can all dream about winning cars, houses and the lottery, but do you think that enables us to really live out our fullest potential? The more we work on ourselves to be free, the more freedom we feel. This is true prosperity!

There is No Final Destination

Be, at a state of peace on your journey. You may have an ultimate goal, but there will always be things to do and places to see. Do not fret about the "things" that arise throughout your journey. If it doesn't bring satisfaction, then it's not meant to be. There will be many areas in your life that you need to look at and this process can't be rushed. So please don't! Just allow the journey to be your main focus for the next while. This is your time to own your true power and become your true self.

You Will Become Fearless

It is my vision that each and every one of us can unleash our inner strength and become fearless in order to make our dreams come true.

It is my vision that each and every one of us takes the stand within our own lives and walks with our heads held high knowing that we have a purpose and a meaning here on this planet.

Your past does not matter. Your present is here and it is in this moment of your life that your future is determined.

As you begin this process, you'll see your life take meaning, take shape and really evolve into what you are truly doing on this planet. I am so excited to really see just how far you are willing to come and embrace all of the beauty that is within you. The meaning and truth that lie not only inside each of us, but through every experience and action that we have created.

If you stick to this program, in 13 weeks you will begin to see and feel this transformation take place within you. You will begin to see your REAL Motivation become your reality, from the time you awaken to the time that you wind down from the day. If you allow yourself to truly LIV, you become the fearless leader in your life.

The choice is yours - take your Ticket and LIV.

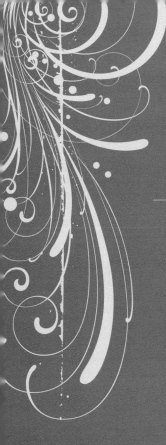

Be Awareness, where there is Awareness there is Knowledge and where there is Knowledge there is WISDOM

The Ticket

CHAPTER FIFTEEN: Get Started With Your New Life

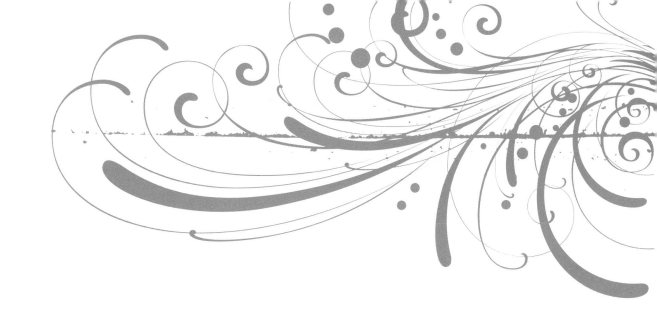

Chapter Fifteen
LIV-
GET STARTED WITH YOUR NEW LIFE

"It is never too late to be what you might have been."

George Eliot

LIV - GET STARTED WITH YOUR NEW LIFE

Inspiration - Rob's Story (39 years of age)

I wanted to include stories of success that I feel could be inspirational to you. It's the stories of Rob and Darlene. Both Rob and Darlene changed their lives when they found the strength to LIV - they uncovered their meaning of life; allowed their desires to become their inspiration; and became present in their vitality. Take their stories as an inspiration and find your own true inner drive to live a transformed life.

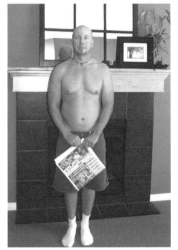

ROB BEFORE

ROB'S STORY:
Why I Started To Get Healthy.
Age: 39

My decision to get healthy was an easy one. I made the decision when my wife called me into the kitchen and informed me I was denied life insurance.

I always believed I was healthy and really never cared what I put in my body or how I treated it. But when your wife comes to you with tears in her eyes because of how unhealthy you've become, it's a real awakening. Then you realize you're not just here for yourself. You have a family that depends on you, that loves and cares for you. Not getting healthy is just being selfish. You get your act together.

My biggest excuses were related to getting to the gym - time constraints or not having the proper equipment. I found that if you use your imagination, everything around you can be used: the park, stairs, benches, rocks and trees - anything you can imagine.

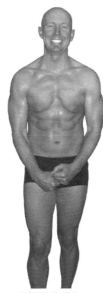

I personally haven't had a gym membership in five years but I do have a mat and ball. This small amount of equipment, along with my own drive and determination, was more than enough to get my mind, body and spirit on track!

Getting healthy was hard, but it got easier and easier as you see and feel the results. One piece of advice I have is get your mind right because when you do, everything just becomes easy. You don't need people to push you. You just need inspiration, which comes from yourself.

ROB AFTER

DARLENE'S STORY:
My Journey.
Age: 44

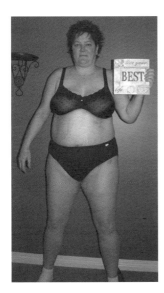

I've always wanted to find true balance in my life but never thought it was possible. When my girlfriend's five-year-old daughter asked me if I had a baby in my belly and I said no, she looked confused and couldn't understand why my belly was so big. No malice, just an honest voice from a child. That was it for me - I cried for hours.

Could I really find happiness daily and still follow my dreams? For years I had been told that's a bunch of hooey. I was eighty pounds overweight and a closet alcoholic - I had to find a way! Learning to be truly honest with myself and looking deep into my spirit, I finally found clarity. Harmony and balance can happen on daily basis if you work hard and start forgiving yourself and forget the past once and for all.

DARLENE BEFORE

liv

It hasn't been an easy journey so far, but trust me, at 44 years old I have never been happier! I quit my job and decided it was time for me to finally be kind to my mind, body and spirit.

Now, six months later and 52 pounds lighter, I continue to follow my path and try to live in the moment and embrace change and all the challenges that face me every day. I now look forward to the future with hope, love and find myself smiling just because. Life is oh so good!

Darlene

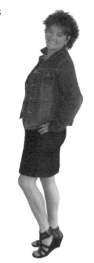

DARLENE AFTER

MY STORY:

It all began...

_____

_____

_____

_____

_____

_____

MY BEFORE

MY AFTER

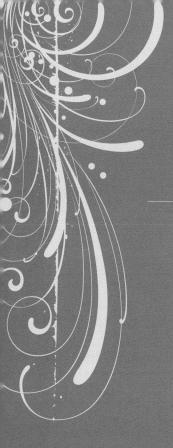

Be Life, where there is Life there is Meaning, and where there is Meaning there is PURPOSE

Resources

CHAPTER SIXTEEN: The Exercise Library

CHAPTER SEVENTEEN: Recipes

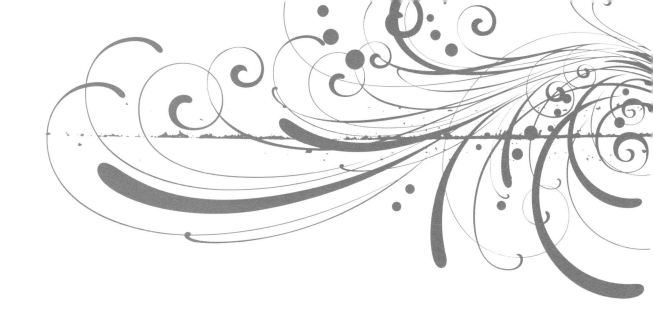

Chapter Sixteen
THE EXERCISE LIBRARY

"You see, you don't get old from age, you get old from inactivity, from not believing in something."

Jack Lalanne

THE EXERCISE LIBRARY

This program consists of exercises that can be done at any time and anywhere with a minimal amount of equipment. Each exercise here in this library is made to challenge you as you become stronger and progress through each level, I have provided modifications so you can change anything within the program.

The more we live within our bodies, and pay attention to them, the more we are living in the moment and the faster we will begin to see and feel the transformation. Each step, each workout, each day is what you need to focus on. It doesn't matter how fast you go or which road you take. It's all about the climb. Focus on the fact that you're taking control of your body and creating a workout regime that gets you excited!

Each exercise is altered to suit three different levels: Bronze, Silver and Gold.

Exercise Modifications

The easiest way to change the intensity of a strength exercise is by changing hand positions. If you feel yourself no longer being challenged by an exercise, try these different hand positions:

- Arms in front of you
- Hand on hips
- Hands behind head
- Arms straight up in the air

Changing the intensity is another way to add variation to your workouts:

- Pace - alternate fast and slow intervals for a certain amount of time
- Changing your grade - lunges up a hill or down
- Change your workout environment - hills or stairs

Contractions – there are three types:

Eccentric: the active lengthening action of a muscle, such as lowering a weight down gently.

Concentric: the active shortening action of a muscle, such as lifting a weight.

Isometric: when a muscle is held for a length of time, such as a wall squat held for thirty seconds to a minute or longer

Program Variations

Circuit: Circuit training develops strength, flexibility, cardiovascular health, coordination and endurance at the same time. It consists of a wide variety of short exercises in one session, with a minimal amount of rest.

Hill training: Taking cardio, lower body or upper body exercises on a hill is a great way to increase its intensity. Run up a hill, do sit-ups facing downwards or do calf raises. Hill training will strengthen your mind, body and spirit.

Interval: Interval training is exercise that consists of spurts of high-energy activity alternated with low intensity or rest. An example of interval training is a period of sprinting followed by a period of light jogging or walking, and so on.

Stair training: Running or lower body exercises done on stairs are great for strengthening your legs and glutes. It's also great for building endurance.

Super sets: Super sets are two different exercises for one particular muscle or group. For example, try doing a set of lunges then super setting with a set of squats, or a chest press followed by push-ups.

Pyramid Sets: Pyramid sets are when you perform a different number of the reps for 5-6 sets. For example: perform push-ups for the following sets and reps. 12-10-8-10-12.

LOWER BODY EXERCISES
Muscle Group - Quads, hamstrings, glutes, hips, thighs and calves

LUNGES (muscles: quads, hamstrings, glutes)
Lunges are one of the most versatile lower body exercises and the best thing about them is you can do them anywhere. Master the form first at the bronze level by putting a foot on an elevated surface, then work your way through the other levels. I would rather you be familiar with your form and feel the movement before you progress.

Bronze: Basic Lunges

Starting Position:

- Stand tall, chest up, shoulders back, core tight
- Place your hands on your hips or have your arms straight out in front of you

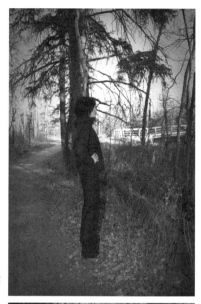

Movement:

- Inhale as you step one foot forward onto a low rock, tree stump or step
- Bend your back knee and drop your hips. Hold for a count of one
- Exhale as you push off the surface through your heel back to starting position
- Repeat and continue on the opposite leg
- Repeat for the number of targeted sets and reps

Watch out for:

- Knees should not extend beyond your toes
- Move straight down into the lunge – do not lean forward
- Chest remains tall, shoulders back and core is activated throughout the movement
- Your breath

Variations:

- Instead of alternating, complete the total number of reps for each leg before you switch
- Change your arm position

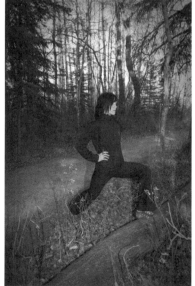

170

Silver: Walking Lunges

Starting Position:

- Stand tall, chest up, shoulders back, core tight
- Place your hands on your hips or have your arms straight out in front of you

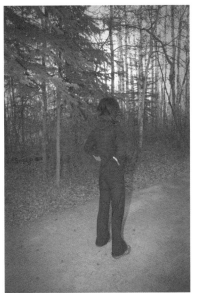

Movement:

- Inhale as you step one foot forward, bend your back knee and drop your hips. Hold for a count of one
- Exhale as you push yourself up through your heel, and take a step forward with your opposite leg, just as if you are walking
- Repeat for the number of targeted sets and reps

Watch out for:

- Posture
- Knees should not extend beyond your toes
- Move straight down into the lunge – do not lean forward
- Core is contracted
- Your breath
- Eyes forward

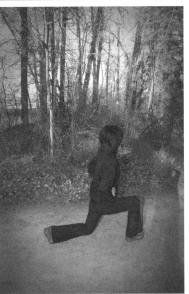

Variations:

- Change your arm position
- Increase your step forward so your back leg is straight
- Increase step forward, with toes pointed outward (you will get a little more inner thigh activation)
- Hold while in the lunge position for a count between one and five

liv

Gold: Uphill Lunges

Starting Position:

- Stand in front of an incline such as a hill
- Stand tall, chest up, shoulders back, core tight
- Place your hands on your hips or have your arms straight out in front of you

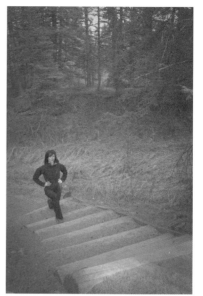

Movement:

- Inhale as you step one foot forward, bend your back knee and drop your hips
- Exhale as you push through your heel and take a step forward as if you are walking
- Repeat for the number of targeted sets and reps

Watch out for:

- Posture
- Knee not over your toes
- Lunge movement is straight up and down
- Core is contracted
- Your breath
- Eyes are forward

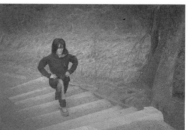

Variations:

- Change your arm or hand position
- Increase your step forward
- Angle your toes outwards to fire up those inner thighs

SQUATS (muscles: hamstrings, quads, glutes)

Squats are a powerful exercise that will help you ignite your inner strength. Starting out at the Bronze level by having something to sit down on will help you feel safe, teaching you how easy it is to find your inner fire to push through to Gold!

Bronze: Touch Squats

Starting Position:

- Stand tall, chest up, shoulders back, core tight with feet hip-width apart
- Stand with a bench or rock behind you

Movement:

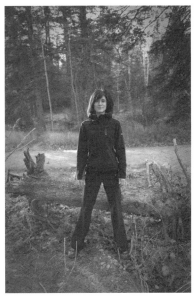

- Inhale as you bend your knees and drop your hips back slightly
- Come down until you feel the surface behind you
- Hold for a count of one
- Exhale as you push through your heels, squeezing your glutes and bringing your hips forward back to the start position in a controlled manner
- Repeat for the number of targeted sets and reps

Watch out for:

- Posture – you may need to bring your shoulders forward slightly for balance, but keep your spine straight
- Knees should not extend beyond your toes
- Core is contracted
- Your breath

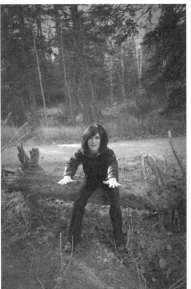

Variations:

- Change your arm or hand position
- Angle your toes outwards to fire up those inner thighs
- Find a lower surface to squat down to touch
- Hold or pulse while in the squat position

Silver: Sumo Squats

Starting Position:

- Stand tall, chest up, shoulders back, core tight
- Feet are wider than shoulder width apart, toes pointed out.

Movement:

- Inhale as you bend your knees and bring your hips back slightly
- Squat until your thighs are parallel with the ground, keeping your weight on your heels. Hold for a count of one
- Exhale as you push through your heels, squeezing your glutes and bringing your hips forward
- Pivot on the ball of your left foot so you are lifting your right leg to turn your body 90 degrees from your original position
- Repeat for the number of targeted sets and reps

Watch out for:

- Posture – you may need to bring your shoulders forward slightly for balance, but keep your spine straight
- Knees should not extend beyond your toes
- Your bent legs should form a 90 degree angle
- Core is contracted
- Your breath

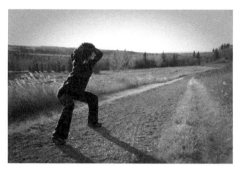

Variations:

- Change your arm or hand position
- Angle your toes outwards to fire up those inner thighs
- Hold a weight or rock above your head
- Hold or pulse while in the squat position

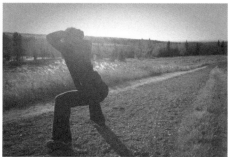

Gold: Jumping Squat

Starting Position:
- Stand tall, chest up, shoulders back, core tight and eyes forward
- Feet are wider than shoulder width, toes pointed forward

Movement:

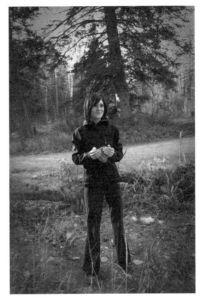

- Inhale as you bend your knees into a squat position. Thighs should be parallel to the ground
- Hold for a count of one
- Exhale as you jump up to extend your legs and then bend them back down into the squatted position
- Repeat for the number of targeted sets and reps

Watch out for:
- Knees should not extend beyond your toes
- Posture
- Exhale on the way up
- Your weight is in your heels

Variations:

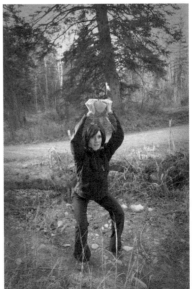

- Change your arm or hand position
- Hold or pulse while in the squat position
- Jump forward or back

liv

STEP-UPS (muscles: quads, hamstrings, glutes)

Step-ups are a fantastic lower body exercise. They work your entire lower body and can easily be done anywhere and at any tempo. Try speeding up your tempo to add a little cardio by increasing your HR. Be aware of how you feel. If it's too hard at Gold with your hands above your head, try placing them on your hips or in front of you. What is most important is that you're using your inner strength to complete this exercise!

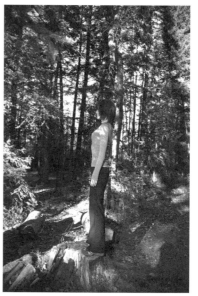

Bronze: Basic step-ups

Starting Position:
- Stand facing stair, step or rock
- Stand tall, chest up, shoulders back
- Feet under hips

Movement:
- Exhale as you lift your right leg and step up, pushing through your right foot
- Inhale and step your left foot back down softly, followed by your right foot
- Alternate with each leg
- Repeat for the number of targeted sets and reps

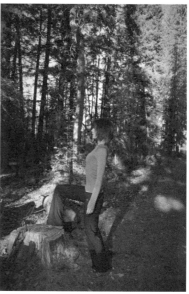

Watch out for:
- Push into your heel as you step up, not the ball of your foot
- Chest is high
- Eyes are forward
- Stand tall when on the top
- Hips are forward

Variations:
- Change your arm or hand position

- Angle your toes outwards as you step up to get those inner thighs
- Change your tempo to a faster pace
- Find a higher surface (keep your knee at or lower than hip level)

Silver: Wider step-ups

Starting Position:

- Stand facing stair, step or rock
- Stand tall, chest up, shoulders back
- Feet under hips

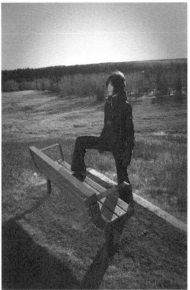

Movement:

- Exhale as you lift your right leg and step up, your toes pointed outwards, your left leg should follow
- Inhale and step your right leg back down softly, followed by your left
- Alternate with each leg
- Repeat for the number of targeted sets and reps

Watch out for:

- Push into your heel as you step up, not the ball of your foot
- Chest is high
- Eyes are forward
- Stand tall when on the top of stair, step or rock
- Hips are forward
- Your breath

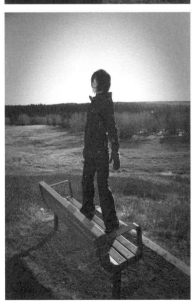

Variations:

- Change your arm or hand position
- Speed it up, or slow it down
- Find a higher step

177

Gold: Kick-back step-ups

Starting Position:

- Stand facing stair, step or rock
- Feet are shoulder width apart
- Stand tall, chest up, shoulders back
- Hands are straight in front of you

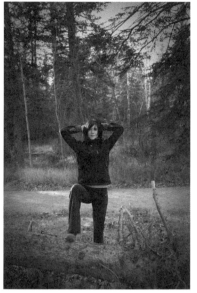

Movement:

- Exhale as you lift your right leg and step up
- Squeeze your left glutes as you kick your left leg behind you
- Hold for a count of one
- Inhale and step your left foot back down softly, followed by your right foot
- Repeat one leg at a time ensuring you lead with the same foot
- Repeat for the number of targeted sets and reps

Watch out for:

- Chest is high
- Eyes are forward
- Hips are forward
- Stand tall when on the top of stair, step or rock
- Squeeze your glutes
- Your breath

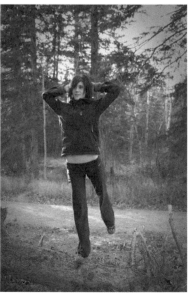

Variations:

- Change your arm or hand position
- Speed it up, or slow it down
- Add an upper body exercise such as a hammer curl

178

ONE LEGGED DIP (muscles: hamstrings, quads, glutes)

You will really feel the intensity with this exercise!

Bronze: Basic One Legged Dip

Starting Position:

- Stand with your back to the stair, step or rock
- Place one foot behind you so your toe is in contact with the surface
- Stand tall, chest up, shoulders back
- Hands should be at your side

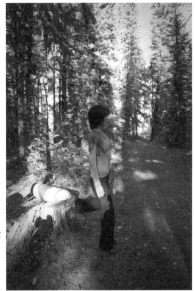

Movement:

- Inhale as you bend your knee, dropping your hips so you are parallel to the floor. Hold for a count of one
- Exhale as you push through your heel to the start position in a controlled manner
- Repeat for the number of targeted sets and reps

Watch out for:

- Ensure you are far enough away from the rock or bench
- You squat deep enough
- Knee not over your toes
- Chest is high
- Eyes are forward
- Your breath

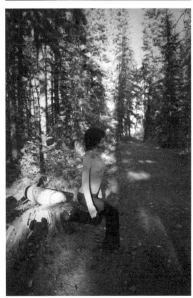

Variations:

- Change your arm or hand position
- Speed it up, or slow it down

liv

Silver: Reverse One Legged Dip With Bicep Curls

Starting Position:

- Stand with your back to the stair, step or rock
- Place one foot behind you so your toe is in contact with the surface
- Place your hands in the handles and your foot under the resistance band in front of you
- Stand tall, chest up, shoulders back

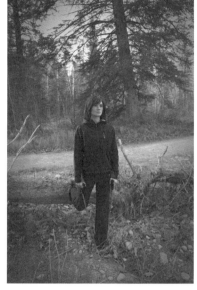

Movement:

- Inhale as you bend your knee, dropping your hips
- While maintaining the squatted position complete a biceps curl
- Exhale as you push through your heel to the start position in a controlled manner
- Repeat for the number of targeted sets and reps

Watch out for:

- Ensure you are far enough away from the stair, step or rock
- Knees should not extend beyond your toes
- Chest is high
- Eyes are forward
- Core contracted to maintain balance
- Your breath

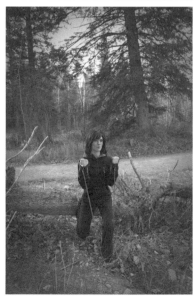

Variations:

- Hold for a count of five
- Speed it up, or slow it down

Gold: Arms Over Head One Legged Dip

Starting Position:

- Stand with your back to the stair, step or rock
- Place one foot behind you so your toe is in contact with the surface
- Stand tall, chest up, shoulders back
- Hands should be straight up in the air

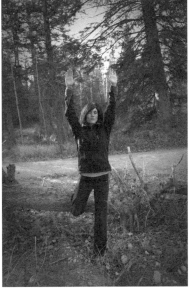

Movement:

- Inhale as you bend your knee, dropping your hips
- Exhale as you push through your heel
- Bringing your pelvis forward squeezing your glutes as you return to the start position in a controlled manner
- Repeat for the number of targeted sets and reps

Watch out for:

- Ensure you are far enough away from the rock or bench
- Knees should not extend beyond your toes
- Chest is high
- Eyes are forward
- Core contracted to maintain balance
- Your breath

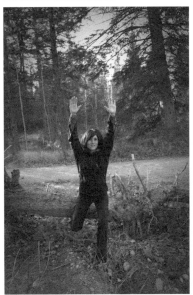

Variations:

- Hold for a count of five to ten
- Speed it up, or slow it down

BRIDGES (muscles: glutes, hamstrings, core)

These are great to really get your glutes and core activated. They are amazing for allowing yourself to focus on your contractions and feel the muscles within you.

Bronze: Basic Bridges

Starting Position:

- Lie on your back with knees bent, feet slightly apart
- Arms are at sides
- Shoulders are pressed into the floor/ground

Movement:

- Exhale as you contract stomach muscles and raise and squeeze buttocks up to a position where the back is straight
- Hold
- Inhale as you squeeze glutes and slowly lower to the start position in a controlled manner
- Repeat for the number of targeted sets and reps

Watch out for:

- Your breath
- Push through your heels
- Squeeze your glutes and contract your core

Variations:

- Hold and squeeze the glutes for 30 seconds

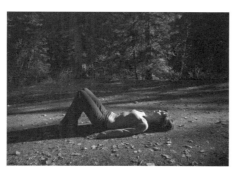
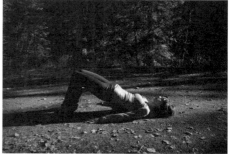

- Pulse for a count of 20
- Change your contraction type

Silver: Elevated Bridges

Starting Position:
- Lie on your back and place both feet on a step or rock
- Your legs should be shoulder width apart.
- Arms are at sides
- Shoulders are pressed into the floor/ground

Movement:
- Exhale as you contract stomach muscles and push through the heels into the rock or step, raising and squeezing your buttocks up to a position where the back is straight.
- Hold for a count of one
- Inhale as you squeeze glutes and lower down slowly to the start position in a controlled manner
- Repeat for the number of targeted sets and reps

Watch out for:
- Your breath
- Push through your heels

Variations:
- Hold the glutes and squeeze for 30 seconds
- Change your contraction type: fast/slow

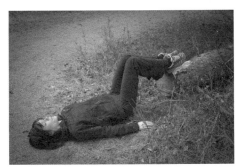 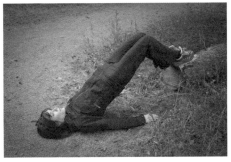

liv

Gold: Crunch Straight-Legged Bridge

Starting Position:

- Lie on your back and place one foot on a rock or step
- Your other leg should be straight in the air
- Hands are at your ears and your shoulders are pressed into the floor/ground

Movement:

- Exhale as you contract your stomach muscles and push through your heels on the step/rock, raising your hips in the air
- Squeeze your glutes and complete an abdominal crunch at the same time
- Hold for a count of one
- Inhale as you slowly lower to the start position in a controlled manner
- Repeat for the number of targeted sets and reps

Watch out for:

- Your breath
- Squeeze your glutes and contract your core

Variations:

- Your hand position
- Hold the glutes and squeeze for 30 seconds while completing 5-10 crunches

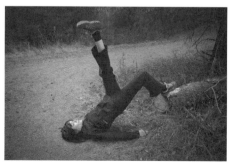 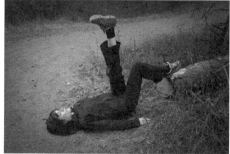

CALF RAISES (muscles: calves)

Calves are a great muscle and sometimes are a muscle that we forget about. Our calves give us the strength to take one step at a time!

Bronze: Walking Calf Raises

Starting Position:

- Stand tall, chest up, shoulders back, facing forward with your hands on your hips or at your side
- Ensure you feel grounded and connected

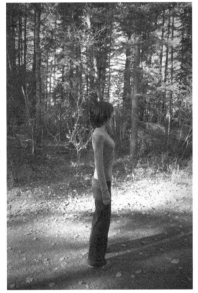

Movement:

- Exhale as you step one foot forward, rolling slowly onto your tiptoes
- Core is activated to ensure your balance
- Lower your heel back to the ground
- Inhale as you walk your other leg forward and complete the same movement
- Repeat for the number of targeted sets and reps

Watch out for:

- Posture
- Your balance – don't go all the way on your tip toes at first if you can't make it
- Core is contracted
- Your breath
- Squeeze your calf muscles

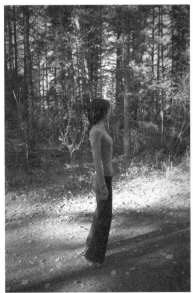

Variations:

- Your hand position
- Your speed of movement

185

Silver: Double Calf Raises

Starting Position:

- Stand with your feet shoulder width apart with only the balls of your feet on the edge of a step
- Stand tall, chest up, shoulders back and core activated
- Hold onto a wall or rail if needed for balance

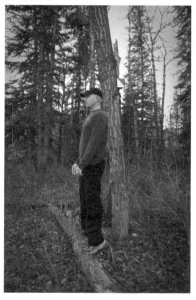

Movement:

- Exhale as you roll onto your tiptoes, contracting your calf muscles
- Hold for a count of one
- Inhale as you drop your heels past the start position in a controlled manner
- Repeat for the number of targeted sets and reps

Watch out for:

- Posture
- Your balance
- Core is contracted
- Your breath

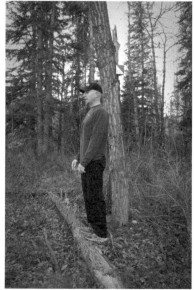

Variations:

- Your hand position
- Your speed of movement
- Perform one leg at a time

Gold: Angled Calf Raises

Starting Position:
- Stand tall on a step with chest high and core activated
- Your feet should be hip width apart
- Place only the ball of your foot on the step
- Your toes should be on an outward angle

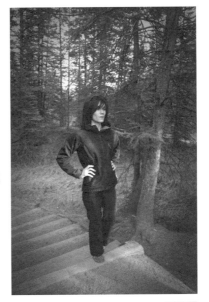

Movement:
- Exhale as you contract your calves by rolling onto your tiptoes
- Hold for a count of one
- Inhale as you slowly lower to the start position in a controlled manner
- Repeat for the number of targeted sets and reps

Watch out for:
- Posture remains tall
- Your balance
- Core is contracted
- Your breath
- Hold on to a wall or rail if you need it for balance

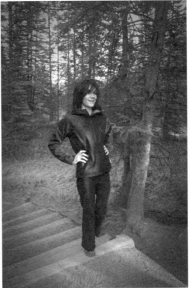

Variations:
- Your hand position
- Your speed of movement
- Perform one leg at a time

UPPER BODY EXERCISES
Muscle Group - Chest, back, shoulders, biceps and triceps

PUSH-UPS (muscles: chest)
Push-ups are great, and there are so many variations of them. What's great about them is that they can be modified to any level.

Bronze: Wall Push-up
Starting Position:
- Stand comfortably away from wall, high counter, stump, or bench (you may have to experiment with distance)
- Put your hands on your chosen surface at shoulder height, hands in line with shoulders

Movement:
- Inhale as you bend your elbows to bring your chest towards the surface
- Hold for a count of one
- Exhale as you straighten your elbows and return to the start position in a controlled manner
- Repeat for the number of targeted sets and reps

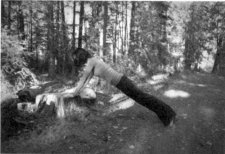

Watch out for:
- Don't lock your elbows
- Ensure you are completing your full range of motion but have your chest come close to the surface
- Hips are in line and core is activated - no belly buttons or bums out!
- Your breath

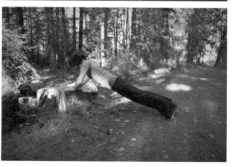

Variations:
- Change your surface; try a lower surface once you have mastered the movement.

Silver: From the Knees

Starting Position:
- Lie face down on the ground with your knees in contact with the floor
- Your hands are placed a little wider than shoulder width apart

Movement:
- Exhale as you lift your body off the ground, squeezing your shoulder blades down and back
- Hold for a count of one
- Inhale as you bend your elbows and slowly return to the start position in a controlled manner
- Repeat for the number of targeted sets and reps

Watch out for:
- Don't lock your elbows
- Ensure you are completing your full range of motion
- Hips are straight and core is activated - no belly buttons or bums out!
- Your breath

Variations:
- Progress to your toes

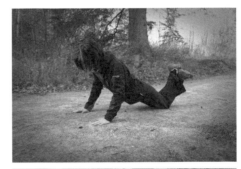

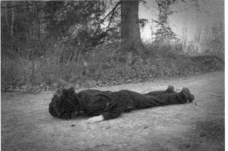

 liv

Gold: From the Toes

Starting Position:
- Lie face down on the floor/ground with your toes in contact with the floor
- Your hands should be in line with your shoulders

Movement:
- Exhale as you lift your body off the floor/ground, squeezing your shoulder blades down and back
- Hold for a count of one
- Inhale as you bend your elbows and slowly return to the start position in a controlled manner
- Repeat for the number of targeted sets and reps

Watch out for:
- Don't lock your elbows
- Ensure you are completing your full range of motion
- Hips are straight and core is activated
- Your breath

Variations:
- Complete your push-ups on a decline
- Try doing them while balancing on one leg

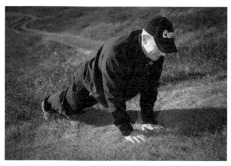 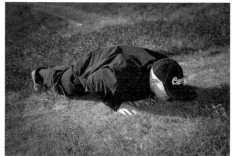

CHEST PRESS (muscles: chest)

Holding your chest high and shoulders back allow you to walk with presence.
When working on your chest think about really owning your uniqueness!

Bronze: The Standing Press

Starting Position:

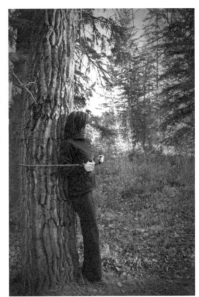

- Find a tree or post and wrap your resistance band around it a few times so it doesn't slide down
- Place your back on the tree and your hands in the band handles
- Ensure you feel balanced and connected to the surface you are on
- Place your arms by your side, elbows bent
- Stand tall, chest high, shoulders back

Movement:

- Exhale as you push forward to straighten your arms - keep elbows soft
- Hold for a count of one
- Inhale as you bend your elbows and slowly return to the start position in a controlled manner
- Repeat for the number of targeted sets and reps

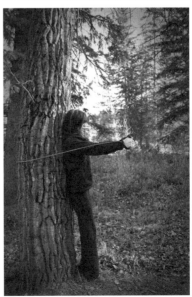

Watch out for:

- Don't lock your joints
- Don't allow your elbows to go back further than your starting position
- Your breath

liv

Silver: The Lying-Down Chest Fly

Starting Position:
- Lie on a surface that you feel secure on, such as a bench or a fallen tree
- Place your resistance band around the object, or have the weights ready in your hands
- Ensure you feel balanced and connected to the surface you are on
- Make a fist with your hands, palms facing upward
- Your arms should be straight to the side

Movement:
- Exhale as you contract your chest by bringing your arms straight to meet over your breast bone, with elbows soft
- Hold for a count of one
- Inhale as you return to the start position in a controlled manner
- Repeat for the number of targeted sets and reps

Watch out for:
- Don't lock your joints
- Don't allow your arms to go back further than your starting position
- Your breath

Variations:
- Change the intensity by changing the resistance
- Change the speed of your contraction or movement

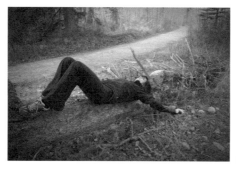
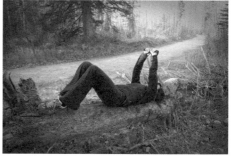

192

Gold: The Lying-Down Chest Press

Starting Position:

- Lie on a surface that you feel secure on, such as a bench or fallen tree
- Place your resistance band around the object or have a weight ready in your hands
- Ensure you feel balanced and connected to the surface you are on
- Hold on to the handles of the band or your weight with your palms facing each other
- Elbows bent at 45 degrees

Movement:

- Exhale as you squeeze your chest and bring your forearms together to meet, keeping your arms straight
- Hold for a count of one
- Inhale as you return to the start position in a controlled manner
- Repeat for the number of targeted sets and reps

Watch out for:

- Don't lock your joints
- Don't go further than the starting position
- Your breath
- Keep your eyes focused and see your hands meet in the middle
- Arms should be taut - no spaghetti arms!

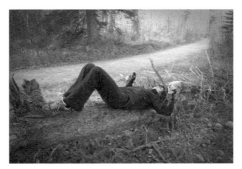

Variations:

- Change the intensity by changing the resistance
- Change the speed of your contraction or movement
- Activate your core by lifting one leg off the surface

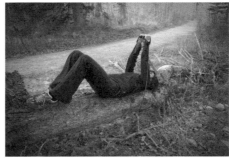

 liv

THE ROW (muscles: back)

Rows are an excellent way to attain alignment for posture. My tip is to imagine that you are squeezing a pencil between your shoulder blades.

Bronze: The Seated Row

Starting Position:

- Sit on the floor with legs extended straight
- Place the centre of your resistance band around the feet, holding one end in each hand
- Be sure the band has some tension when arms are extended forward
- Keep your posture tall, core tight, shoulders back and down

Movement:

- Exhale and pull elbows close to body until maximum tension is reached, or hands are close to body
- Hold for a count of one
- Inhale as you return to the start position in a controlled manner
- Repeat for the number of targeted sets and reps

Watch out for:

- Posture remains tall
- Your focus is on squeezing your back
- Breathe

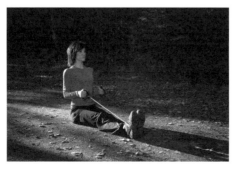 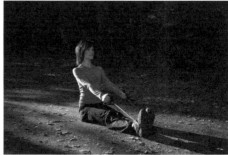

Silver: The Bent Over Row

Starting Position:

- Stand with slightly bent knees, torso bent forward at waist, straight back
- If you are using a resistance band, stand on it
- Grasp band handles or weights so your palms are facing each other
- Core is activated

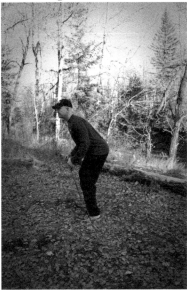

Movement:

- Exhale as you contract your back muscles and pull the band up, with your elbows brushing your rib cage
- Hold for a count of one
- Inhale with arms extended as you return to the start position in a controlled manner
- Repeat for the number of targeted sets and reps

Watch out for:

- Posture
- You are leaning over far enough
- Eyes are looking forward
- Core is activated
- Your spine is straight and chest is tall

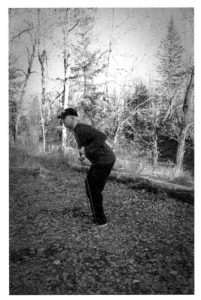

liv

Gold: Leaning Row

Starting Position:

- Place band around a tree
- Face the tree and hold onto the handles of the band with your palms facing each other
- Stand tall with your back straight and core tight
- Ground your feet and lean back so band is taut

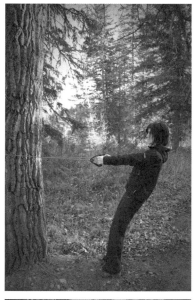

Movement:

- Exhale as you contract your back muscles, brushing your elbows against your rib cage
- Hold and squeeze your back muscles
- Inhale with arms extended as you return to the start position in a controlled manner
- Repeat for the number of targeted sets and reps

Watch out for:

- Eyes straight ahead
- Core is activated
- Your spine is straight and chest is tall
- Keep your shoulders back and in alignment
- Don't lock your joints

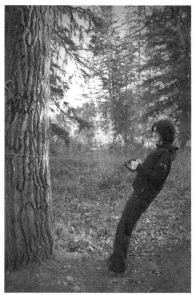

WALL ANGELS (muscles: rhomboids, back)

These are great for you to work on your posture. It may look simple but it's a killer. If it feels too easy, your form might be off.

Bronze: Wall Angel

Starting Position:

- Stand with your back against a surface
- Your feet should be four inches from the wall with buttocks, spine and head against the surface
- Raise arms up along wall with elbows parallel to the ground

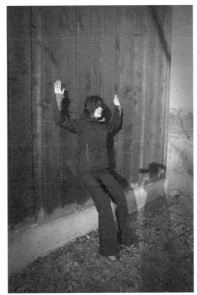

Movement:

- Contract your back muscles (isometric contraction)
- Hold this position for a count of 15
- Breathe
- Inhale with arms extended as you return to the start position in a controlled manner
- Repeat for the number of targeted sets and reps

Watch out for:

- Your arms, hands and shoulders need to remain in contact with the wall at all times
- The small of your back should be pressed into the wall. You can check by placing your hand at your lower back. If there is space, flex your pelvis forward.

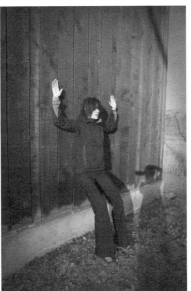

liv

Silver: The Half Angel

Starting Position:

- Stand with your back against a surface
- Your feet should be four inches from wall with buttocks, spine and head against the surface
- Raise arms up along wall, toes should be level, elbows bent

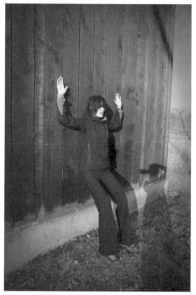

Movement:

- Exhale as you bring hands towards each other overhead (still against wall)
- Hold for a count of five
- Inhale as you lower to the start position in a controlled manner
- *If any part of your arms or hands come away from the wall, that is your end point. Your goal is to meet your hands overhead but your range of motion is limited to where you find you are leaving the surface*
- Repeat for the number of targeted sets and reps

Watch out for:

- The small of your back should be pressed into the wall. You can check by placing your hand at your lower back. If there is space, flex your pelvis forward.
- Use slow, controlled movements

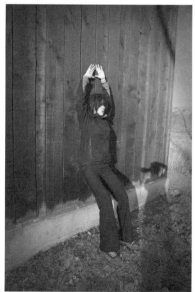

198

Gold: The Full Angel (when you've perfected the Half Angel form)

Starting Position:

- Stand with your back against a surface
- Your feet should be four inches from wall with buttocks, spine and head against the surface
- Raise arms up along wall, toes should be level, elbows bent

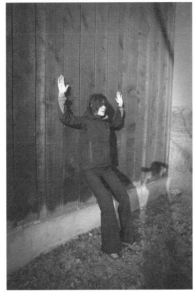

Movement:

- Exhale as you bring hands towards each other overhead (still against wall)
- Hold for a count of one
- Inhale as you bend your elbows and lower your arms to try to meet your elbows to your rib cage
- *If any part of your arms or hands come away from the wall, that is your end point. Your goal is to meet your hands overhead but your range of motion is limited to where you find you are leaving the surface*
- Hold for a count of one
- Repeat for the number of targeted sets and reps

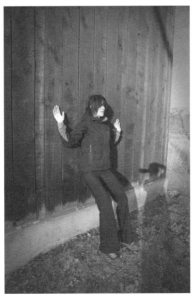

Watch out for:

- The small of your back should be pressed into the wall. You can check by placing your hand at your lower back, if there is space, flex your pelvis forward
- Your breath

liv

SHOULDER RAISES (muscles: deltoids)

Shoulders are a great muscle to work and take the stress away from your body!

Bronze: Seated Earth Raiser

Starting Position:

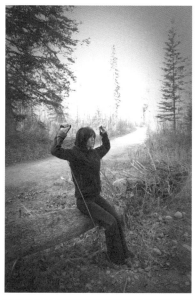

- Sit on a surface
- Place band under feet and grasp with both hands
- Raise arms to shoulder level
- Palms facing forward
- Keep your core tight

Movement:

- Exhale as you contract your shoulder muscles to bring your hands to meet overhead
- Hold for a count of one
- Inhale as you return to the start position in a controlled manner
- Repeat for the number of targeted sets and reps

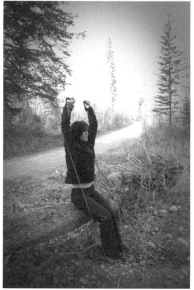

Watch out for:

- Chest remains tall
- Your breath
- Eyes remain forward
- Your arms don't go past start position

Silver: Standing Earth Raiser

Starting Position:

- Stand tall with your arms bent to 45 degrees to your side
- Place band under feet and grasp with both hands
- Contract core by tilting your pelvis forward

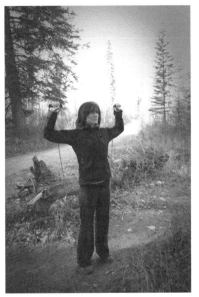

Movement:

- Exhale as you contract your shoulders, pulling the band in a straight position meeting hands over head (palms facing forward)
- Pause for a count of one
- Inhale as you return to the start position in a controlled manner
- Repeat for the number of targeted sets and reps

Watch out for:

- Chest remains tall
- Your breath
- Eyes remain forward

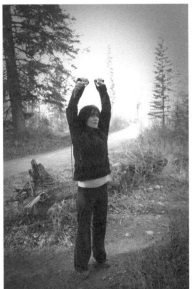

liv

Gold: Front and Side Earth Raiser

Starting Position:

- Stand tall on the band, core tight, hands grasping handles
- Tuck your pelvis to prevent your lower back from swaying

Movement:

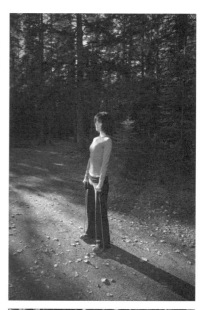

- Exhale as you bring your arms straight out in front of you so your arms are parallel to the floor/ground
- Hold for a count of one
- Inhale as you slowly return to the start position in a controlled manner
- Exhale as you raise your arms to the side this time, parallel with the floor/ground
- Hold for a count of one
- Repeat for the number of targeted sets and reps

Watch out for:

- Chest remains tall
- Your breath
- Eyes remain forward
- Slow controlled movement
- Full range of motion

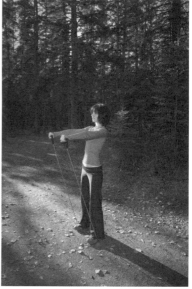

TRICEP DIPS (muscles: triceps)

Toned triceps are a top concern for women, and the good news is you can see the results of this exercise very quickly!

Bronze: Standing Tricep Extension

Starting Position:

- Step on one end of your resistance band and grasp the other end in both hands behind head
- Lower hands down, behind your head, with elbows pointing up
- Inhale as you lower

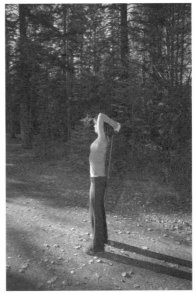

Movement:

- Exhale and slowly extend arms straight above head
- Hold for a count of one
- Elbows must remain stationary and as much in line with shoulders as your flexibility allows
- Inhale as you slowly return to the start position in a controlled manner
- Repeat for the number of targeted sets and reps

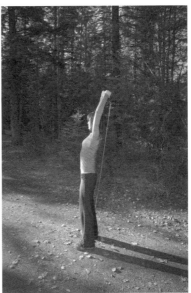

Watch out for:

- Chest remains tall
- Your breath
- Eyes remain forward
- Elbows remain stationary

liv

Silver: Bent Leg Tricep Dip

Starting Position:

- Sit on the edge of a chair, or tree stump that is about chair height to the ground
- Put your hands beside your hips, holding onto the front edge of chair
- Scoot buttocks forward off chair and have legs straight (or knees bent to make it easier)

Movement:

- Inhale and bend your elbows back while you lower your buttocks towards floor/ground
- Hold for a count of one
- Exhale as you straighten your arms and push yourself back up to the start position in a controlled manner
- Repeat for the number of targeted sets and reps

Watch Out for:

- Your breath
- Keep your elbows pointed back, not to the side
- Don't lean too far out from the chair; your back should slightly touch the chair throughout the movement
- Keep your shoulders back, not rounded

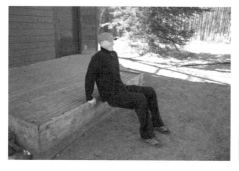 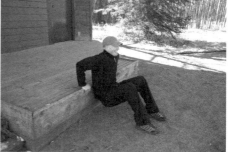

Gold: Straight-leg Tricep Dip

Starting Position:

- Sit on the edge of a chair, or tree stump that is about chair-height to the floor/ground
- Put your hands beside your hips, holding onto the front edge of chair
- Scoot buttocks forward off chair and extend both legs out in front

Movement:

- Inhale and bend your elbows back, lowering your buttocks towards floor/ground
- Hold for a count of one
- Exhale as you extend and push yourself back up to the start position in a controlled manner
- Repeat for the number of targeted sets and reps

Watch Out for:

- Your breath
- Keep your elbows pointed back, not to the side
- Don't lean too far out from the chair; your back should slightly touch the chair throughout the movement
- Keep your shoulders back, not rounded

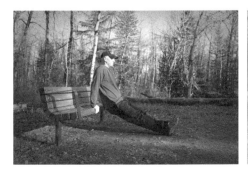 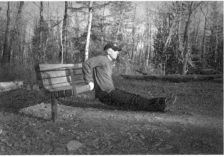

liv

BICEP CURLS (muscle: biceps)

Toned biceps are great for both men and women - who doesn't like toned arms?

Bronze: Basic Curls

Starting Position:

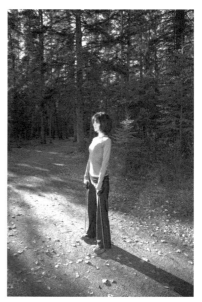

- Stand on the centre of your resistance band, the handles each hand with palms facing up
- Chest tall, shoulders back, core tight
- Elbows are stationary at your sides

Movement:

- Exhale as you bring band/weight up towards shoulders
- Hold and squeeze your biceps for a count of one
- Inhale without locking elbows as you slowly return to the start position in a controlled manner
- Repeat for the number of targeted sets and reps

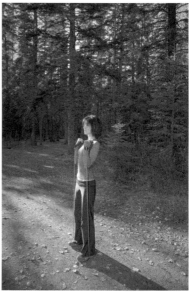

Watch out for:

- Chest remains high, shoulders back
- Your breath
- Don't lock elbows
- Don't sway back and forth
- Slow controlled movements

206

Silver: Hammer Curls

Starting Position:

- Stand on the centre of your resistance band, one end in each hand
- Grasp the handles so your thumbs are pointing upwards, palms facing each other

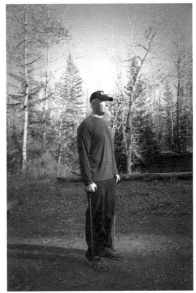

Movement:

- Exhale as you curl, bringing your hands to your shoulders
- Hold for a count of one
- Inhale without locking elbows as you slowly return to the start position in a controlled manner
- Repeat for the number of targeted sets and reps

Watch out for:

- Chest remains high, shoulders back
- Your breath
- Don't lock elbows
- Don't sway back and forth
- Slow controlled movements

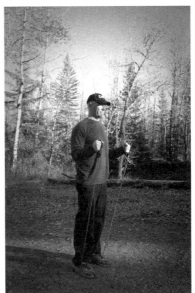

Variations:

- You can increase the intensity by adjusting the band resistance/weights
- Try tucking elbows on an angle into your hip area

Gold: Twenty-ones

Starting Position:
- Stand on the centre of your resistance band, one end in each hand
- Grasp the handles so your palms are facing each other

Movement:

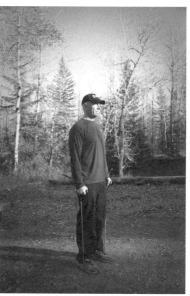

- Exhale as you curl, bringing your hands parallel to the floor (half way)
- Hold for a count of one
- Inhale, return to starting position without locking elbows
- Repeat for a count of seven
- Begin another set of curls, now starting from the halfway mark and finishing at the shoulder
- Repeat for a count of seven
- For the last seven reps, complete full bicep curls - all the way down and all the way up
- For these last seven, tuck your elbows into your hip area and angle outwards
- Repeat for the number of targeted sets and reps

Watch out for:
- Chest remains high, shoulders back
- Your breath
- Don't lock elbows
- Don't sway back and forth
- Slow, controlled movements

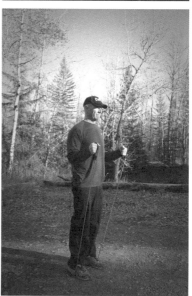

Variations:
- You can increase the intensity by adjusting the band resistance/weights

CORE EXERCISES
Muscle Group - Abdominals, lower back and obliques

SUPERMANS (muscle: lower back)

These are great as they allow you to really feel your back. Just remember to engage your core!

Bronze: Basic Superman

Starting Position:

- Lie on your stomach with your elbows bent, hands by shoulders
- Contract your core - pull your belly button off the floor/ground

Movement:

- Exhale as you squeeze your glutes and lift your chest off the floor/ground slightly
- Inhale as you return to the start position in a controlled manner
- Repeat for the number of targeted sets and reps

Watch out for:

- Push through your thighs and calves to support the movement and prevent back pain
- Your breath
- Keep your core tight throughout the movement
- Neck - allow your head to come up naturally with the movement

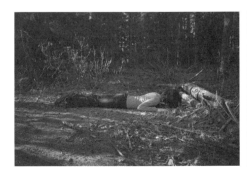
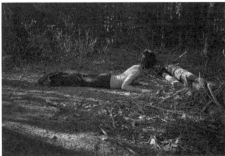

liv

Silver: Intermediate Superman

Starting Position:

- Get on all fours - hips over knees and hands under shoulders
- Contract your core

Movement:

- As you exhale, squeeze your glutes, raise and reach one arm and the opposite leg at the same time
- Hold for a count of one
- Inhale as you return to the start position in a controlled manner
- Repeat for the number of targeted sets and reps

Watch out for:

- Keep your spine straight - no saggy backs!
- Core is tight
- Don't raise your head - look at the ground
- Slow, controlled movements
- Your breath

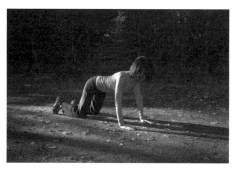 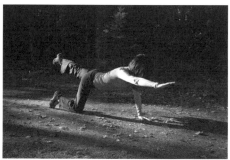

Gold: Flying Superman

Starting Position:

- Lie flat on your stomach
- Place your arms straight out in front of you
- Contract your core

Movement:

- As you exhale, squeeze your glutes as you lift both arms and legs in the air
- Hold for a count of three
- Inhale as you return to the start position in a controlled manner - ensuring your legs and arms barely touch the surface
- Repeat for the number of targeted sets and reps

Watch out for:

- Your breath
- Core is activated throughout the entire movement

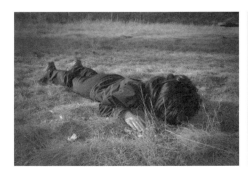 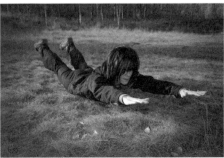

SIT-UPS (muscles: core)

I think each and every one of us should be able to do a sit up. Just keep working on them and you will be driven by the progress you will make. Imagine there is a cord attached to your belly button helping you with each rep!

Bronze: Basic Sit-up

Starting Position:
- Lie on your back, with knees bent
- Have someone hold your toes or tuck them under a chair or table
- Put your arms straight in front of you

Movement:
- Exhale as you contract abdominals, raising your head, neck and back off floor up to a comfortable position
- Hold for a count of one
- Inhale as you return to the start position in a controlled manner
- Repeat for the number of targeted sets and reps

Watch out for:
- If you are having trouble, try decreasing the angle of your legs
- Lying on an incline with your head on the high end will help with your form
- Your breath
- Don't make jerky movements or pull your head up with your hands
- Chin should be tucked slightly

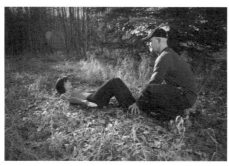
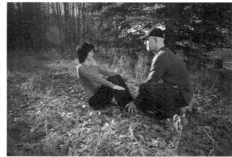

Silver: Sit-up

Starting Position:

- Lie on your back, with your knees bent
- Cross your hands over your chest or have them touching your ears

Movement:

- Exhale as you contract abdominals, raising your head, neck and back off floor up to a comfortable position
- Hold for a count of one
- Inhale as you return to the start position in a controlled manner
- Repeat for the number of targeted sets and reps

Watch out for:

- Feet should remain in contact with the floor
- If you are having trouble, just tuck your toes
- Your breath
- Don't make jerky movements or pull your head up with your hands

Variations:

- Try different arm movements, such as a quick twist with a left-right punch as you complete each sit-up

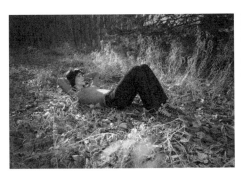 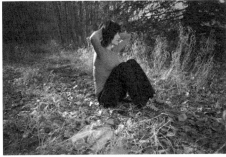

Gold: Advanced sit-up

Starting Position:

- Lie on your back on an inclined surface, your feet facing up the incline
- Knees bent and legs at a 45 degree angle
- Cross your hands over your chest or have them touching your ears

Movement:

- Exhale as you contract abdominals, raising your head, neck and back off floor up to a comfortable position
- Hold for a count of one
- Inhale as you return to the start position in a controlled manner
- Repeat for the number of targeted sets and reps

Watch out for:

- Chin should remain tucked
- Your breath
- Don't make jerky movements or pull your head up with your hands
- Core is activated throughout the entire movement

Variations:

- Try different arm movements, such as a quick twist with a left-right punch as you complete each sit-up

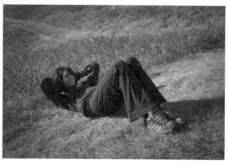 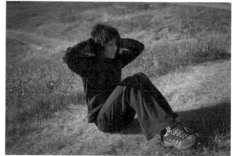

CRUNCHES (muscles: rectus abdominals)

Crunches are great as they allow you to really feel the burn and you can feel them working right away. Remember to activate your core by pushing your lower back in to the floor/ground.

Bronze: Basic Crunch

Starting Position:

- Lie on floor/ ground with knees bent, feet flat on floor/ground and tucked under a rock or chair
- With hands clasped together behind your ears, elbows out to the sides, press your lower back into the floor/ground

Movement:

- Exhale through your mouth as you contract abs to bring head, neck, and shoulders off floor/ground (think about bringing your face closer to the ceiling)
- Inhale as you return to the start position in a controlled manner
- Repeat for the number of targeted sets and reps

Watch-out for:

- Breath
- Don't make jerky movements or pull your head up with your hands
- Support yourself by pressing your lower back into the floor/ground

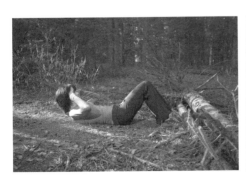 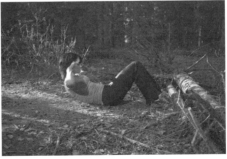

Silver: The Strong Core Crunch

Starting Position:

- Lie on the floor/ground with knees bent
- Your arms are straight above your head

Movement:

- Exhale through your mouth as you contract abs and lift to bring head, neck, and shoulders off floor/ground (think about bringing your face closer to the ceiling)
- Hold for a count of one
- Inhale as you return to the start position in a controlled manner, maintaining the contraction
- Repeat for the number of targeted sets and reps

Watch out for:

- Your breath
- Support yourself by pressing your lower back into the floor/ground
- Keep your neck straight; tuck chin and look up

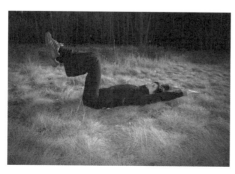 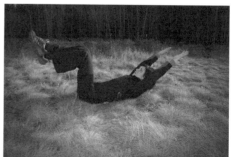

Gold: The V-Crunch

Starting Position:

- Lie on your back with your hands overhead and your feet stretched out in front of you
- Contract your core

Movement:

- Exhale as you lift your legs and arms at the same time to form a V-shape with your body
- Hold for a count of one
- Inhale as you return to the start position in a controlled manner
- Repeat for the number of targeted sets and reps

Watch out for:

- Your breath
- Be controlled throughout the movements

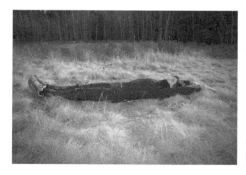
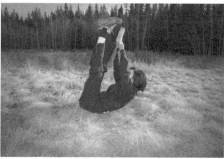

PLANK (muscle: core)

These may seem hard at the beginning as you are working your upper body as well, but keep with it and you will notice how much more power you'll have!

Bronze: Plank from Knees

Starting Position:
- Lie face down on the floor/ground and fold your arms against your side
- Make a fist with your thumbs facing upwards
- Your forearms should be flat on the floor/ground
- Your elbows should be under your shoulders
- Core is tight

Movement:
- Exhale as you raise your upper body off the floor/ground, balancing on your knees and forearms
- Take slow deep breaths
- Hold for as long as you can, keeping core tight

Watch out for:
- Ensure your back is straight
- Pelvis tilted - no bottoms out
- Your breath

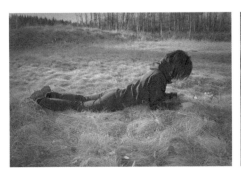 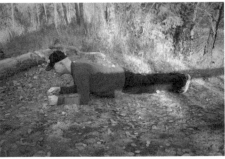

218

Silver: Straight-arm Plank

Starting Position:

- Lie face down on the floor/ground and fold your arms against your side
- Make a fist with your thumbs facing upwards
- Your forearms should be flat on the floor/ground
- Core is tight

Movement:

- Exhale as your straighten one arm at a time, so you are balancing on your palms and toes
- Inhale as you lower the same way you came up.
- Right arm up, left arm up. Right arm down, left arm down
- Repeat for the number of targeted sets and reps

Watch out for:

- Ensure your back is straight
- Pelvis is tucked
- Core is tight
- Keep your hands under your shoulders
- Your breath

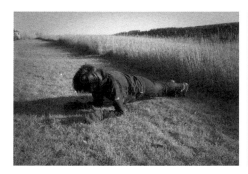 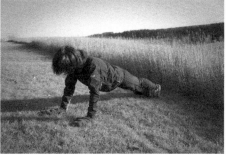

Gold: Inchworm Plank

Starting Position:
- Lie face down on the floor/ground and fold your arms against your side
- Lift your body off the floor/ground and balance on your hands and toes

Movement:
- Exhale as you contract your core
- Walk your toes forward 4-6 steps
- Inhale and walk your hands forward 4-6 steps
- Perform a single row with each arm and then continue the movement
- Repeat for the number of targeted sets and reps

Watch out for:
- Your breath
- Core remains engaged throughout the entire movement.
- You need to have the core and upper body strength to perform this exercise without compromising the form

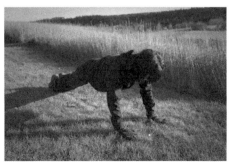 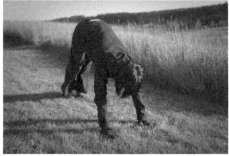

REVERSE LEG LIFT (muscle: abdominals)

Most of us forget about our lower abs, and this exercise is excellent for getting them stronger. A strong core is the key to a strong back!

Bronze: Basic Leg Lift

Starting Position:

- Find a hard surface to sit on, such as a rock, bench or chair
- Place your hands at either side of your hips
- Start with your buttocks further back and then work your way closer to the edge

Movement:

- Exhale as you contract your core and lift your legs off the ground as far as you can
- Hold for a few seconds
- Inhale as you lower your legs almost to the ground and repeat
- If you are unable to perform this exercise with your legs straight, perform it with bent legs
- Repeat for the number of targeted sets and reps

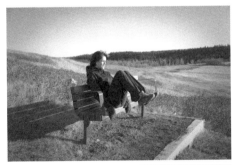

Watch out for:

- Your back should be straight, your core tight and you should be leaning back a little
- Chest is tall, eyes are forward
- Engage your abdominal muscles
- Your buttocks should be on the edge of the seat

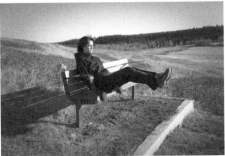

Variations:

- Bring your knees to your chest and out to each side

Silver: Lying-down Leg Lift

Starting Position:

- Lie on your back with your legs straight
- Hold on to a tree, a doorway or the ankles of someone standing at your head

Movement:

- Exhale as you contract your core, raising your legs vertically from the floor/ground
- Inhale as you slowly lower your legs back down almost to the floor/ground
- Repeat for the number of sets and reps

Watch out for:

- If you find this too challenging with your legs straight, bend them at the knees
- Engage your abdominal muscles and not your back

Variations:

- Add a little obliques by lifting to either side

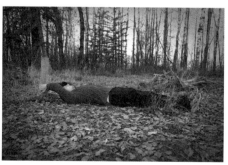 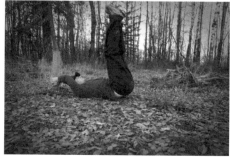

Gold: Advanced Leg Lift

Starting Position:

- Lie on your back with your legs straight
- Hold on to a tree, a doorway or even the ankles of someone standing at your head

Movement:

- Exhale as you contract your core, raising your legs vertically from the floor/ground
- Once your legs are up, lift your buttocks off the floor by pushing your heels to the ceiling
- Inhale as you slowly lower your legs back down ensuring your feet don't touch the floor/ground
- Repeat for the number of targeted sets and reps

Variations:

- Raise your legs to either side
- Add a few pulses while your buttocks are lifted

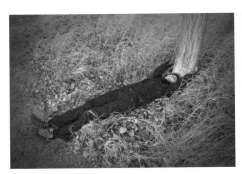
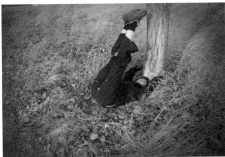

SIDE PLANK (muscles: obliques)

With this exercise, you will feel your entire core activated.

Bronze: Knee Side Plank

Starting Position:

- Lie on your side with your knees bent at a 45 degree angle
- Your elbow should be under your shoulder and your forearm in contact with the floor/ground
- Place your other hand on the floor in front of you for support
- Double check to see if your body is straight, if not, your hips are probably out of alignment. Tilt your pelvis

Movement:

- Exhale as you raise your hips off the floor/ground, balancing on your forearm and knees
- Hold for as long as you can while breathing deeply
- Contract your core even tighter and breathe
- Repeat for the number of sets and reps

Watch out for:

- Your body needs to be straight with neck in alignment
- If you are feeling pain in your shoulder or your arm, ensure that you are in proper alignment with your elbow under your shoulder
- Navel tucked into your spine
- Your breath
- Pelvis tucked

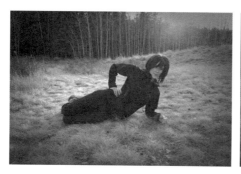 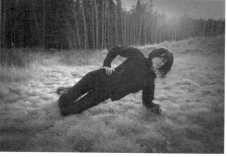

Silver: Toes Side Plank

Starting Position:

- Lie on your side with your legs straight
- Your elbow should be under your shoulder and your forearm in contact with the floor/ground
- Place your other hand on your hip
- Double check to see if your body is straight, if not, your hips are probably out of alignment. Tilt your pelvis

Movement:

- Exhale as you raise your hips off the floor/ground, balancing on your forearm and sides of your feet
- Hold and breathe deeply
- Contract your core even tighter and lift your hips further up
- Inhale as you return to the start position in a controlled manner
- Repeat for the number of sets and reps

Watch out for:

- Your body needs to be straight; pelvis tucked
- If you are feeling pain in your shoulder or your arm, ensure that you are in proper alignment with your elbow under your shoulder
- Slow deep breaths
- Core tight

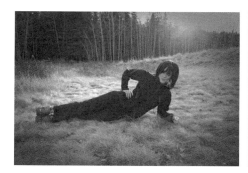
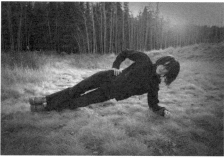

liv

Gold: Twist Side Plank

Starting Position:
- Lie on your side with your body straight
- Your elbow should be under your shoulder and your forearm in contact with the floor/ground
- Make a fist with thumb facing up
- Place your other hand on your hip to balance
- Double check to see if your body is straight, if not, your hips are probably out of alignment. Tilt your pelvis inward

Movement:
- Exhale as you raise your hips off the floor/ground, balancing on your forearm and sides of your feet
- When you feel balanced, extend your other arm into the air
- With your arm extended, bring it down in front of your chest reaching behind your body (twisting motion)
- Hold for a count of one
- Exhale as you return to the start position in a controlled manner
- Repeat for the number of targeted sets and reps

Watch out for:
- Your breath
- Core contracted through out the entire movement.
- Hips in alignment
- When returning to the starting position, ensure your arm does not go past your shoulder; it may throw you off balance

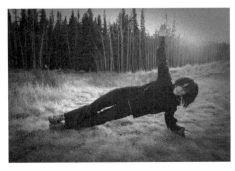 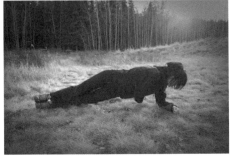

V-TWIST (muscles: abdominals, obliques)

This is an exercise that allows you to feel the burn. By changing up the tempo you will definitely feel an increased intensity.

Bronze: Basic V-twist

Starting Position:
- In a seated position with feet on the floor/ground
- Lean back slightly; this will contract your core
- Your chest should be nice and tall, shoulders back
- Bring your hands together in front of you; envision you are holding a rock or ball

Movement:
- Exhale as you twist your upper body from side to side, as if you are moving the ball to touch the floor/ground on either side of hips
- Your pace should be controlled, a count of one for each movement
- Exhale as you return to the start position in a controlled manner
- Repeat for the number of targeted sets and reps

Watch out for:
- Your breath
- If you are finding it too difficult with your legs at 90 degrees, decrease knee angle by moving your heels further away from your buttocks
- Shoulder blades are back and spine is straight

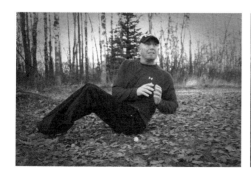 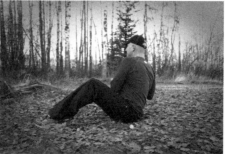

Silver: Weighted V-twist

Starting Position:

- In a seated position with your feet on the floor/ground
- Lean back slightly; this will contract your core
- Your chest should be nice and tall, back contracted
- Hold your weight or rock in front of you

Movement

- Exhale as you twist your upper body to place the rock or weight beside your hip
- Inhale as you continue from side to side
- Your pace should be controlled, a count of one for each movement
- Repeat for the number of targeted sets and reps

Watch out for:

- Shoulder blades are back and spine is straight
- Keep your feet in contact with the floor/ground
- Core remains engaged
- Feel yourself anchored to the floor/ground through your glutes.
- Your breath

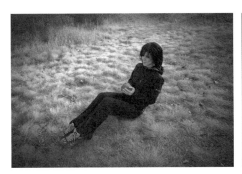 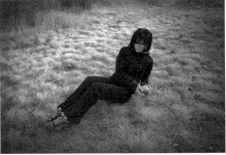

Gold: Leaned Back V-twist

Starting Position:

- In a seated position with your feet on the floor/ground
- Lean back slightly; this will contract your core
- Your chest should be nice and tall, back contracted
- Hold your weight or rock in front of you.

Movement:

- Exhale as you slowly lean back towards the floor/ground as you twist with your body from side to side, touching the weight to the floor/ground on either side of you
- Count to five on the way down
- Inhale and count back up to five on the way up
- Repeat for the number of targeted sets and reps

Watch out for:

- Keep your chest high, shoulder blades down and back
- Your breath
- Your speed while performing the exercise should be smooth and controlled
- Your core is activated throughout the entire movement.

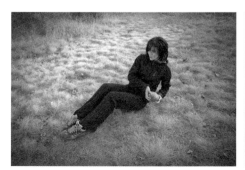 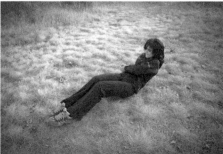

 liv

ADVANCED TO INTERMEDIATE FULL BODY EXERCISES

Full body exercises are great when you want a quick but high intensity workout.

Please make sure that you and your body are ready for the exercises listed here. You don't want go overboard and run the risk of hurting yourself. Don't allow your mind to take over; this is an excellent opportunity for you to tune into your body and see what it tells you. Keep your heart rate in mind as well, so you don't over-exert yourself.

Walking sumo with spice!
Start walking and when you are in the squat position, try:
- Overhead shoulder press
- Chest press
- Triceps extension
- Add a quick punch to either side

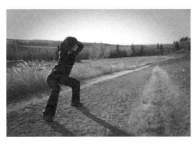 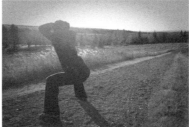

Walking lunges with spice!
Start walking and when you are in the lunge position, try:
- Overhead shoulder press
- Chest press
- Triceps extension
- Add a quick punch to either side

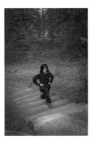 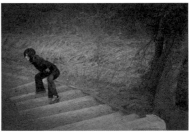

Step-ups

Find your favourite spot with a step or
bench and try:

- Overhead shoulder press
- Chest press
- Triceps extension
- Add a kick to the side, front or
  back - just watch your balance
- Add a quick punch to either side

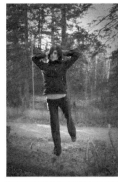
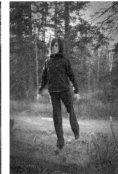

The killer sumo

While doing the sumo exercise, hold a
rock or weight overhead. Feel that burn
- see how long you can hold it. Drop
the rock first!

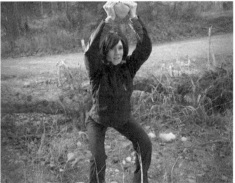

Jack meets sumo

We all know jumping jacks - why not
combine it with a sumo?

- Complete a jumping squat but
  jump all the way up and touch your
  hands overhead, just like a jumping
  jack

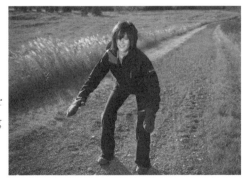

Workout Clean

Short on time? If you need to clean your house and get your workout in at the
same time - do both!

- Put your HR monitor on and get moving
- Alternate cleaning a floor and doing five sets of step-ups
- While vacuuming, perform walking lunges to get around. Stay in an isometric
  sumo squat while you vacuum under your table.

liv

- Take a break and do some dips on a chair, then turn over and do push-ups from a table or the floor
- Hey why not add a few sets of stairs at the same time.

CARDIO

Anything can be considered cardio. It's all about getting your blood pumping. Get moving and see your heart rate climb on the monitor. Ensure you know what your target zone is and work from there!

Here are some of my favourites for cardio:

Step-ups
Find a step and get stepping

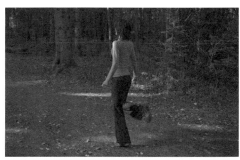

Bum kicks
Do them walking or even running. Just watch your form.

High knees
Place your hands out in front of you at a level as a target for how high to lift your legs. Change it up with your level of lift and speed or try them on an angle.

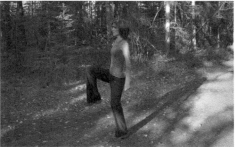

Shuffles
Stand with your feet wider than shoulder width apart and shuffle to the side. It might take a bit to get the form down, but when you do, they are fun. Just remember to do the other side as well.

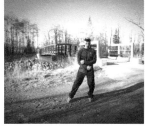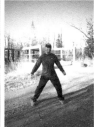

232

Mountain climbers

Begin on all fours, hands under shoulders. Then jump one foot forward so your knee is under your chest, then the other. Alternate back and forth and see if you can get some speed!

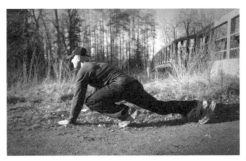

Burpies

On the spot, jump up with arms straight overhead then jump down to bring hands down beside feet and then kick both legs out behind, touching the ground with your feet. Then jump forward, feet between arms. Jump up with arms in the air and repeat.

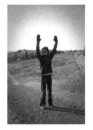 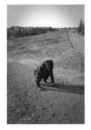 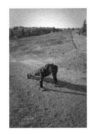 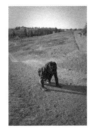 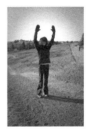

Running

If you are not a runner, just start slow. Try 3:1 - walk for three minutes and run for one minute. Be aware of your form. Program page 121

Hill training

Run a figure eight on the hill or do all of your strength training exercises on an incline

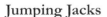

Jumping Jacks

Really gets your heart rate up.

Skipping

It never seemed this hard when we were kids!

liv

Stairs

This is a killer workout! Alternate singles and doubles, wide leg singles and doubles

Dancing

Get ready and rock it out! All you closet rock stars, Latin dancers or ballerinas; here is your chance to shine! Listen to music and move!

STRETCHES

Stretching is something that many people leave out of their exercise routine or rush through. I promise that if you allow this time to relax, unwind, and reflect your body will love you for it. I have included a few yoga poses as well. They are not only great for stretching your body but they help you to unwind!

How to properly stretch:

- Stretch muscles that you worked that day

- Don't over stretch - it should feel good and not painful

- Hold for at least 20-30 seconds

- Make smooth movements – no bouncing or jerking

- Breathe slowly and deeply

- On the exhale reach further into the stretch, follow the rhythm of your breath.

- Be in your body, quiet your mind and use this time to live from within.

LOWER BODY STRETCHES
Muscle Groups - Calves, hamstrings, quads, and glutes

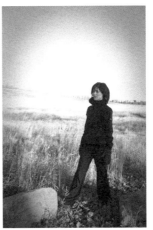

Toes Up Stretch
- Place your toes onto something like a rock or a step
- Slightly lean forward
- You should feel the stretch in your calf
- If you need more of a stretch, tighten your core and lean forward slightly
- Take long, slow, deep breaths
- Hold for at least 20-30 seconds
- Switch and repeat on the opposite side

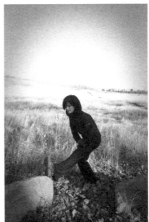

Hamstring Stretch
- Find a rock and place one heel on it
- Gently lean forward and feel the stretch
- Pull your hips back to feel more intensity
- Breathe deeply
- Hold for 20-30 seconds
- Switch and repeat on the opposite side

Standing Quad Stretch
- Stand tall, chest up, shoulders back
- Bend your leg so your heel is pointed towards your buttocks
- Reach back and with your hand, grab your toes
- Feel the stretch in your quad - add a little more by tilting your hips forward
- Breathe deeply
- Hold for 20-30 seconds
- Switch and repeat on the opposite side

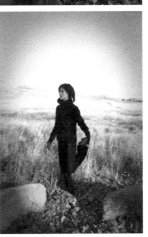

liv

Tree Glute Stretch

- Find a tree and hold on with both hands
- Place one foot on the opposite knee - you should feel the stretch in your glute right away
- Hold on to the tree and lean slightly back and feel the stretch through your entire body
- Breathe deeply
- Hold for 20-30 seconds
- Switch and repeat on the opposite side

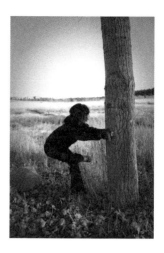

One Seated Hamstring Stretch

- Sit tall and stretch one leg out in front of you, with the other leg bent
- Inhale as you reach forward to touch your toes, feel the stretch in your hamstrings
- If you are tight as most people are, you might find that your knee comes up. If this happens, slowly ease into your lean
- Breathe deeply
- Hold for 20-30 seconds
- If you find that one leg is tighter than the other, repeat on that side.
- Switch and repeat on the opposite side

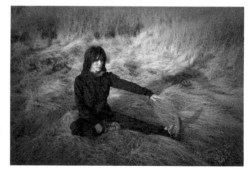

Leaning Quad Stretch

- Sit nice and tall - chest is high, shoulders back, core is activated
- Bend knee and slide leg back to your side. See picture
- Place your forearms on the ground behind you for support
- You may feel the stretch here. If you want more, lean back slightly and tilt your pelvis forward

- Breathe deeply
- Hold for 20-30 seconds
- Switch and repeat on the opposite side

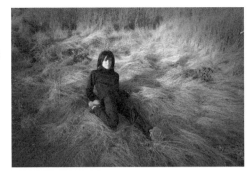

Leg Back Glute Stretch

- Lie on your back, lift your left leg and bend at the knee
- Place the right heel on your left knee
- Hold on to the elevated leg behind the knee
- Feel the stretch
- To increase the stretch, pull your knee close to your chest
- Breathe deeply
- Hold for 20-30 seconds
- Switch and repeat on the opposite side

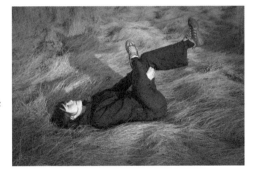

Feet First Stretch

- Sit tall - chest is high, shoulders are back
- Core is tight
- Bending knees, keeping them close to floor, bring soles of feet together and hold onto your toes
- With each exhale; try allowing your knees to come closer to the floor/ground, feel stretch in your inner thigh
- Breathe deeply
- Hold for 20-30 seconds

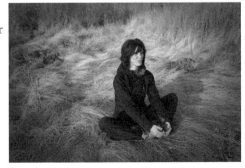

liv

Twist Glute Stretch

- Sit tall with your legs straight in front of you
- Chest is tall, shoulders are back, and core is tight
- Bend your right leg and cross it over your straight left leg, keeping the right knee close to your chest (your right foot should be close to your hip)
- Brace your arm on the outside of your right knee and twist, looking in the opposite direction
- Feel the stretch in your glutes and back
- Keep your chest high and shoulders back
- Breath deeply
- With each exhale; twist your chest a little further
- Hold for 20-30 seconds
- Switch and repeat on the opposite side

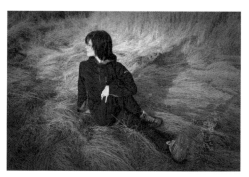

UPPER BODY STRETCHES

Muscle Groups - Chest, back, triceps and biceps

Tree Chest Stretch

- Find a tree, a post or even a wall
- Place right hand on wall and push against the surface to twist yourself the opposite way
- You should feel the stretch in your chest and shoulders and arms
- Breathe deeply and hold for 20-30 seconds
- Switch and repeat on the opposite side

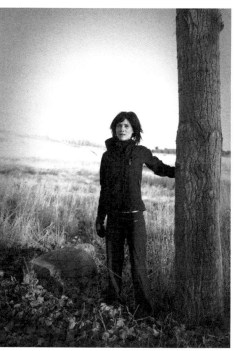

Thumbs Down Stretch

- Stand tall, with your shoulder blades down and back, core tight and hips aligned
- Bring one arm behind you and point your thumb to the ground
- You should feel the stretch in your biceps
- Breathe deeply and hold for 20-30 seconds
- Switch and repeat on the opposite side

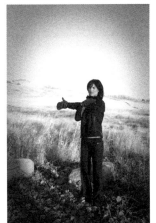

Shoulder Cross Stretch

- Sit or stand tall, shoulders back, chest high, core tight
- Bring your arm across your chest
- Ensure your arm is nice and straight - no spaghetti arms!
- With the other hand, put pressure on the extended elbow to feel the stretch
- Breathe deeply and hold for 20-30 seconds
- Switch and repeat on the opposite side

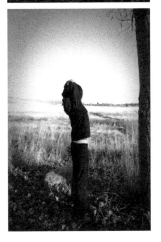

Overhead Tricep Stretch

- Stand tall, shoulders back, chest high, core tight
- Raise your arms over your head, bending one of them at the elbows
- With the other hand, press back against the elbow and feel the stretch
- Breathe deeply and hold for 20-30 seconds
- Switch and repeat on the opposite side.

liv

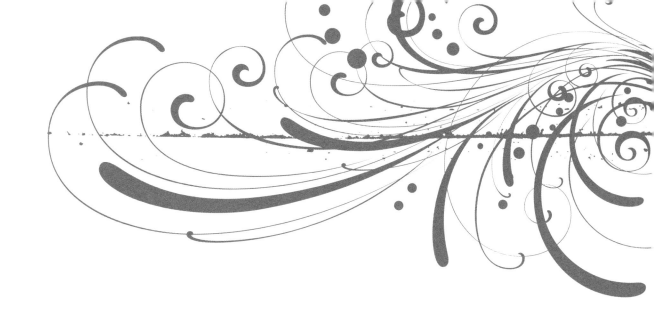

Chapter Seventeen
RECIPES

"As the days grow short, some faces grow long.
But not mine. Every autumn, when the wind turns cold
and darkness comes early, I am suddenly happy.
It's time to start making soup again."

Leslie Newman

RECIPES
Tips for busy lifestyles

We all have busy lives. I know for myself and my family we need quick, easy, nutritionally-dense food that not only satisfies my time limits but is also great tasting. These recipes are simple, affordable and the whole family will love them!

Cooking is fun and I think the whole family should be involved. You can even have designated family members cook on certain nights. For example: Mom cooks Mondays, Wednesdays and Fridays. Dad can cook Tuesdays, Thursdays and Sundays and the kids do Saturday nights. Cooking is and should be a team effort, from deciding on meals, to buying groceries, to washing and prepping and then to actual cooking. The more everyone chips in, the easier and enjoyable mealtime becomes.

In order to completely prepare for your "Nutritional Lifestyle", you're going to need some tools. First and foremost, depending on your schedule, you're probably going to have to pack a few lunches. Invest in an insulated lunch bag that will keep your cold foods cold until lunch. A few different Tupperware containers are perfect to hold your lunch as well. I like the medium sized ones; this way you can put your whole meal with a side salad in one. Snacks are perfect for smaller containers.

I've provided some recipes you can try out during the 13 weeks and beyond, balanced with carbs, proteins and fats. These are some of my family favourites and I hope you enjoy them too. Remember, recipes are very versatile. You can substitute any of the ingredients that you may not like for another. If you aren't a fish person, try the same recipe with your favourite meat or poultry. If you don't like broccoli, try cauliflower! The most important thing here is that you are taking the time to consciously become aware of this "Nutritional Lifestyle".

I have also signified the carbs, fats and proteins in each recipe with a **C**, **F** and **P.**

Remember servings sizes will vary depending on your needs. Adjust when necessary.

Enjoy!

BREAKFAST
Chocolate Oat Breakfast Cookie

These are great to make on the weekend and keep in the freezer to pop in your lunch for either breakfast or a snack when you are on the run. You might even think you are cheating by having a cookie in the morning. Your kids will love them too!

Prep Time: 10 mins
Cook Time: 20 mins
Serves: 10

> 1 cup whole-wheat flour
> 1 tsp baking soda
> 2 eggs whites
> 1/3 cup safflower oil
> 1¼ cup applesauce
> 1/2 cup brown sugar, honey or brown rice syrup
> 2 tsp vanilla
> 3 cups oats
> 1 package fat free chocolate pudding
> 2 cups cottage cheese (blended in blender/ food processor)
> 1/4 cup chopped nuts (walnuts, almonds, etc.)
> 1/2 cup chocolate chips

C: oats and whole wheat flour **P:** cottage cheese **F:** oil and nuts

- Preheat oven to 350 degrees F.
- Mix all dry ingredients together, then all wet ingredients. Combine the two.
- Place on greased baking sheet in ¼ cup size drops.
- Flatten with a fork and top with nuts.
- Bake for 15-20 minutes.
- Cool and keep refrigerated.

Blueberry Hazelnut Pancakes

Who doesn't like pancakes? These freeze exceptionally well. Toss them in the toaster and you have breakfast in minutes!

Prep Time: 7 mins
Cook Time: 10 mins
Serves 2

4 egg whites
1 cup oats
1/2 cup cottage cheese
1 tsp baking soda
1 tsp vanilla
4 tbsp ground hazelnuts
cinnamon to taste
1/2 cup fresh or frozen blueberries

C: oats and berries **P:** cottage cheese/egg whites **F:** hazelnuts

- Place first five ingredients in a blender and combine.
- Spray a skillet with low-fat spray and heat on medium.
- Pour batter into pan in servings and make pancakes.
- Top with fresh blueberries or create a berry sauce (page 248).

The Perfect Omelet Wrap

Omelets are great for Sunday mornings or if you have a little extra time in the morning to read the paper. It might be even quicker if everything is prepped and ready in the fridge!

Prep Time: 5 mins
Cook Time: 5 mins
Serves 1

3-4 egg whites
3 green onions (chopped)
1/2 green pepper (sliced)
1/2 red pepper (sliced)
2 tbsp grated cheese
1 tbsp milk
salt and pepper and maybe a few herbs of your choice
2 slices of whole grain, sprouted grain bread or a whole-wheat wrap

C: bread **P:** eggs **F:** cheese

- In a non-stick frying pan sauté green onions and peppers until onions become translucent. Remove from pan.
- Beat eggs; add milk, salt and pepper. Pour into same pan as onions and peppers.
- Cook on medium heat until eggs are half cooked. Place the veggie mixture over eggs and add cheese. I like to use a lid to help it along the way.
- When cooked: eggs are set. Flip one side over..
- Serve with toast as a sandwich or a whole-wheat wrap topped with green onions and tomatoes.

Get Moving Morning Smoothie

Smoothies are great as a quick and easy breakfast when you're on the go. They even work as snacks. They are very versatile and you can add any fresh or frozen fruit that you love!

Prep Time: 5 mins
Cook Time: 2 mins
Serves 1

1 cup frozen berries (your choice) blueberries ,strawberries, black berries
1 scoop protein powder
1/2 cup water, juice, milk or yogurt-depending on what you like
1-2 cups ice
2 tbsp flax seed oil

C: berries **P**: protein powder **F**: flax seed oil

- Blend all together in a blender and enjoy!

Vanilla Cinnamon French Toast

Here is one that the kids will love to help with. When children help in the kitchen, it not only builds confidence but this is also an excellent time to share and spend quality time with them.

Prep Time: 5 mins
Cook Time: 5 mins
Serves 2

4 egg whites
3 tbsp 1% milk
2 tbsp ground flax seeds
4 slices whole grain/sprouted grain bread
1 tsp vanilla
cinnamon

Toppings:
1 cup fresh or frozen berries
4 tbsp chopped walnuts

C: bread **P:** eggs **F:** walnuts

- Mix egg whites and milk together.
- Add vanilla and cinnamon.
- Soak bread in egg mixture.
- Place in nonstick frying pan and cook until both sides are golden brown.
- Top with a little syrup, applesauce, fresh berries or berry syrup made from heated or crushed berries with a little honey or agave nectar, and a touch of vanilla.

Toasted Walnut Raisin Oatmeal

When you are in a rush, this is great. Use quick oats and cook them in the microwave. Add the rest, stir and away you go!

Prep Time: 2 mins
Cook Time: 4 mins
Serves 1

1/2 cup oatmeal
1 scoop plain or vanilla protein power
2 tbsp chopped walnuts
1 tbsp raisins
1 tsp vanilla
dash cinnamon

C: oats **P:** protein powder **F:** walnuts

- Cook oatmeal as per package directions. Microwave is quick!
- Add a scoop of protein powder and top with walnuts and raisins. A little cinnamon is good too.
- Depending on your taste buds and your protein powder, you may need to add a little sweetness. Try topping with a little honey or brown rice syrup.

Tiger Power Cereal

This cereal is quick and easy, and there's something magical about your child taking pride in eating a cereal they helped you make. This is a great snack for school or in the afternoon topped with a dollop of yogurt.

Prep Time: 10 mins
Cook Time: 25-30 mins
Serves 10-15

1 cup oats

1 cup kamut puffs (these cereals can all be found in your health food section)

1 cup corn puffs

1 cup millet puffs

1 cup slivered almonds

1/2 cup hemp seeds

1 cup raisins

Coating:

3/4 cup peanut butter (natural or regular)

1 tsp vanilla extract

3/4 cup honey or agave nectar or other sweetener

1/3 cup cocoa (optional)

C: grains **P:** hemp seeds **F:** sunflower seeds, peanut butter

- Preheat oven to 325 degrees F.
- In a big bowl, mix first five ingredients together and set aside.
- In a saucepan, combine coating ingredients until melted.
- Toss over cereal mixture.
- Place on large baking sheet and bake for 15-20 minutes.
- Let cool, add raisins, and place in an airtight container.
- Store on the grain shelf in your pantry.

250

LUNCH
Apple Chicken Salad Pita

This is a great easy lunch. If you don't want to fill the pita, toast it instead and have it as a chicken salad pita dip with chips.

Prep Time: 5 mins
Cook Time: 0 mins
Serves 1

    1 cooked chicken breast cubed
    2 tbsp chopped red onion
    1 tbsp low fat mayonnaise
    1/2 apple diced
    3 strawberries diced
    1/2 whole wheat pita
    alfalfa sprouts or chopped lettuce
    2 tbsp toasted almonds
    salt and pepper to taste

C: pita **P:** chicken **F:** mayonnaise/almonds

- Place cubed chicken in a bowl.
- Add chopped onion, apple, strawberries, salt, pepper and mayonnaise. Mix.
- Place in the pocket of a pita and top with sprouts or lettuce, and toasted almonds.
- Serve with a side salad and enjoy.

Chicken Quinoa Cranberry Spinach Salad

If you are a salad person as I am, you will love this one. If you don't like cranberries, toss some strawberries or oranges in instead.

Prep Time: 7 mins
Cook Time: 0 mins
Serves 1

1 leftover cooked chicken breast, cubed

1/2 cup cooked quinoa

2 tbsp dried cranberries

2 cups spinach

2 tbsp walnuts

2 tbsp chopped red onion or more if you prefer

C: quinoa **P:** chicken **F:** walnuts

- Cook quinoa according to package directions and allow to cool.
- On a bed of pre-washed spinach, place chicken, quinoa, cranberries, red onion and walnuts.
- Serve with your favourite vinaigrette.

Veggies and Chips with Garlic Dip

I love this one, there is just something about having veggies and dip for lunch! You can always make extra dip and use it as a topping for other meals throughout the week.

Prep Time: 10 mins.
Cook Time: 10 mins.
Serves 2

1 cup cottage cheese

1 cup yogurt, low fat plain

2-4 garlic cloves, crushed

1/3 cup chopped parsley

1 tsp onion, chopped fine (a cheese grater is handy for this)

4 tbsp chopped walnuts

2 whole-wheat wrap

sprinkle of paprika

4-5 cups of your favourite veggies

C: whole wheat wraps **P:** cottage cheese **F:** walnuts

- Preheat oven to 350 degrees F
- Blend cottage cheese with yogurt, garlic, parsley and onion.
- Top with walnuts, sprinkle of paprika and let sit.
- Cut wrap into wedges with a pizza slicer.
- Sprinkle garlic powder and salt over cut wrap
- Bake for seven minutes. Flip and bake for another three minutes.
- Wash and chop your veggies and enjoy!

Dijon Mustard Turkey Breast on Rye with side Salad

Add lots of veggie toppings to have a plate filled with colour.

Prep Time: 5 mins
Cook Time: 0 mins
Serves 1

palm size serving of lean roasted deli turkey breast

2 slices rye bread

2 thin slices low fat cheese

tomatoes, sliced

1 green onion, sliced

1-2 tsp dijon mustard

salt and pepper

C: rye bread **P:** turkey **F:** cheese

- Spread mustard on bread.
- Add the turkey, tomatoes, onions and lettuce.
- Sprinkle salt and pepper over the toppings, to taste.
- Serve with a side salad.

254

Sundried Tomato and Basil Chicken Salad

Sundried tomato and fresh basil are an excellent combination, so why not try it on a salad?

Prep Time: 5 mins
Cook Time: 0 mins
Serves 1

1 cooked chicken breast, thinly sliced

1/3 cup sliced sundried tomatoes (find in the produce section)

1-3 tbsp walnuts pieces

1/4 cup green onions, chopped

1/3 cup fresh basil (chopped)

2 cups romaine lettuce

2 slices of whole wheat/sprouted grain bread

2 tbsp parmesan cheese

C: bread **P**: chicken **F:** Parmesan cheese

- Place chopped chicken, sundried tomatoes, onions and walnuts on bed of lettuce and top with Parmesan cheese. Top with low-fat sundried tomato dressing.
- Toast bread, cut a garlic clove in half and rub over warm toasted bread.

DINNER
Almond Savory Breaded Chicken and Yam Fries

Why not try breading your chicken with something different? Crushed walnuts are good here too.

Prep Time: 15 mins
Cook Time: 40 mins
Serves 4

4 skinless boneless chicken breasts

2-4 yams, depending on size

2-3 cups mixed veggies such as cauliflower, broccoli, carrots, beans

1-2 minced garlic cloves

salt and pepper to taste

Breading:

1/4 cup slivered almonds or almond crumbs

2 tbsp savory

2 egg whites, beaten

C: yams **P:** chicken **F:** almonds

- Pre-heat oven to 375 degrees F.
- Place egg whites in a bowl, lightly beat.
- Lightly coat each breast with beaten egg whites and roll in slivered/crushed almonds and savory.
- Place chicken on a non-stick baking pan.
- Cook chicken for approximately 30-35 minutes (ovens may vary).
- Peel and cut yams into thick french fry size pieces and lightly coat with olive oil.
- Toss cut yams with garlic powder and a little bit of savory (if desired).
- Place in oven and bake for 35 minutes, turning every 10 minutes.
- Steam veggies and serve on the side.

Dill Salmon, Wild Rice and Mango Avocado Salad

Have a gourmet meal at home in less than an hour. You can also use a cedar plank to cook your salmon on the barbecue.

Prep Time: 20
Cook Time: 40 mins
Serves 4

    4 salmon steaks

    2 cups uncooked wild rice

    1 large mango (chopped)

    4 cups arugula or mixed greens

    1/2 cups thinly sliced red onion

    1/4 cup sliced avocado

    1/4 cup toasted slivered almonds

    1/2 cups fresh dill (chopped)

C: wild rice **P:** salmon **F:** almonds/avocado

- Preheat oven to 350 degrees F.
- Prep and cook rice as per directions.
- Place salmon on a non-stick baking sheet and top with chopped dill.
- Peel and chop mango, place half on salmon. Save the rest for salad.
- Bake salmon for 20-30 minutes.
- Place mango slices, avocado slices, toasted almonds and onion slices on a bed of arugula.
- Serve with a low-fat vinaigrette and enjoy.

Teriyaki Beef Stir Fry on Whole Wheat Egg Noodles

Stir-fries are quick and easy.. If you are running low on time just add a package of frozen stir fry veggies that you find in the freezer section.

Prep Time: 20 mins
Cook Time: 15 mins
Serves 4

8-10 ounces sirloin beef

1 tsp olive oil

1 red onion (sliced)

4 peppers (sliced)

3 -5 garlic cloves, chopped or minced

2-3 tsp soy sauce

1/4 cup teriyaki sauce (look for low sodium)

salt and pepper to taste

4 cups whole wheat noodles

C: egg noodles **P:** sirloin beef **F:** olive oil

- Place garlic cloves in a non-stick pan, adding beef slices and onions.
- Cook on med-high heat for about 10 minutes, stirring often.
- Prep noodles as per directions.
- Add chopped peppers, salt and pepper, soy sauce and teriyaki sauce, to your beef about 2-4 minutes before pasta is cooked.
- Cover and cook until vegetables are steamed, stir often.
- Serve over noodles.

Barbecue Chicken Pita Pizza with Fresh Garden Salad

It's so quick and easy, your whole family will think it took hours to prepare!

Prep Time: 10 mins
Cook Time: 15 mins
Serves 4

4 whole wheat pitas

2 boneless, skinless chicken breasts, uncooked

1/4 cup barbecue sauce

1 red onion (sliced)

2 red or green peppers

2-3 garlic cloves

1/4 cup low-fat mozzarella

Salad:

4 cups of washed lettuce or spinach

2 cups of your favourite veggies

top with your favourite low fat dressing or vinaigrette dressing

C: Pita **P:** chicken **F:** low-fat mozzarella cheese

- Preheat oven to 350 degrees F.
- Slice chicken into bite size pieces along with onion and peppers.
- Dice or mince garlic.
- Sauté chicken and garlic until partially cooked, add onions, peppers, salt and pepper.
- Cook until done, meat is no longer pink.
- Add barbecue sauce to meat and vegetables.
- Spread all ingredients over pita.
- Shred mozzarella and cover entire pita.
- Bake for 10-15 minutes until heated throughout and cheese has melted.
- Serve with side salad.

Chili

This is a great staple to have as a Ticket Meal. It freezes well, so make extra and place it in a freezer bag. When you need a meal quick, place the bag in a sink filled with water until thawed then heat it up!

Prep Time: 5 mins
Cook Time: 35 mins
Serves 4

1 lb lean ground beef or lean ground turkey

2 tbsp olive oil

1 onion, chopped

3 garlic cloves, minced

2-3 cans kidney beans

2 cans whole or stewed tomatoes

1 tbsp cumin (more if you like)

salt and pepper to taste

C: kidney beans **P:** lean ground beef **F:** sour cream and olive oil

- In a large pan, sauté ground beef with onions and garlic cloves over med-high heat until onions are translucent.
- Add salt and pepper.
- Add the remainder of the ingredients.
- Simmer on low heat for 30-45 minutes.
- Top with thinly sliced green onion and a dollop of fat free sour cream and side salad.

260

Beef Quesadilla

You will love this one - you might even think you're cheating! You can substitute chicken for beef to give it a different flavour.

Prep Time: 10 mins
Cook Time: 15 mins
Serves 4

1 lb beef sirloin strips
1 red small onion, sliced
3 garlic cloves, minced
2-3 green peppers, sliced
2 tbsp soy sauce
4 whole wheat wraps
1/2 cup low-fat shredded cheese
low fat sour cream

C: wraps **P:** beef **F:** olive oil, sour cream

- Preheat oven to 400 degrees F.
- Coat a frying pan with low-fat cooking spray and heat to med-high.
- Add garlic and red onion and sauté for a few minutes, until onions are translucent.
- Add beef sirloin strips and cook, stirring, for 10 minutes.
- Add green peppers and soy sauce. Sauté until beef is cooked.
- Place beef mix on half of the wrap.
- Top with cheese, then fold wrap over.
- Bake in the oven for about 7-10 minutes.
- Serve with low fat sour cream, salsa and a side salad.

liv

Basil Tomato Chicken on Spaghetti Squash

Spaghetti squash is an excellent alternative to pasta.

Prep Time: 15 mins
Cook Time: 30 mins
Serves 4

    4 whole boneless, skinless chicken breasts

    2 spaghetti squash

    2 cans stewed tomatoes or eight fresh tomatoes

    3 garlic cloves

    1 onion, chopped

    1 pepper, chopped

    3 tbsp fresh basil, chopped (or more)

C: spaghetti squash **P:** chicken **F:** parmesan cheese

- Preheat oven to 375 degrees F.
- Place chicken in pan and top with stewed tomatoes, garlic, onion, peppers and fresh basil.
- Cut spaghetti squash in half and clean out seeds.
- Top squash halves with salt and pepper and cover with foil.
- Bake both chicken and squash in the oven for 30-35 minutes.
- Top chicken with a dash of fresh basil and a little Parmesan cheese.
- Using a fork dig out squash- will come out with spaghetti like consistency.
- Place chicken breast over the spaghetti squash and serve with a side of your favourite salad.

Turkey Burger Pita

Burgers are a classic. You can always make extra and freeze them, or roll them into meatballs and use them in your favourite pasta dish.

Prep Time: 10 mins
Cook Time: 25 mins
Serves 4

1 lb ground turkey breast
2 garlic cloves, crushed
1 tbsp Italian seasoning
1 small onion, chopped
1 egg white
1/2 cup of oats
1/4 cup of ground flax seeds
salt and pepper to taste

C: whole wheat pita **P:** ground lean turkey breast **F:** flax seed

- Preheat oven to 350 degrees F.
- Place ground turkey in a bowl.
- Add garlic, seasoning, chopped onion, egg whites and oats.
- Form into patties.
- Coat with ground flax seeds.
- Bake or grill for 30-40 minutes.
- Serve in a whole-wheat pita with the toppings, you can even wrap up with lettuce.
- Serve with a side of veggies and low-fat dressing for a side dip. Ranch works well here.

Topless Lasagna

That's right - you don't need to give up lasagna!

Prep Time: 15 mins
Cook Time: 45 mins
Serves 8

1 lb extra lean ground beef

1 large onion, chopped

1-2 garlic cloves, chopped

1 tsp garlic powder

1-2 tbsp cumin

1 jar tomato sauce

9 whole wheat/rice/kamut lasagna noodles

1/4 cup parmesan cheese or low-fat mozzarella cheese

C: noodles **P:** beef **F:** cheese

- Pre-heat oven to 350 degrees F.
- In a pan, cook beef with spices and sauce.
- Cook pasta and drain.
- In a non-stick baking dish, layer noodles, meat sauce and cheese (2 layers).
- Top with remaining cheese.
- Bake for 40-45 minutes.
- Top with just a little more cheese and serve with your favourite side salad.

SNACKS

Here are some low fat treats that will make you think you're cheating, but remember the serving size!

Blueberry Upside Down Cheesecake

Even if you're not a fan of cheesecake, you will love this one!

Prep Time: 5 mins
Cook Time: 0 mins
Serves 2

   1 cup cottage cheese

   1-2 tbsp fat free vanilla pudding

   1 tsp vanilla

   2 tsp graham cracker crumbs

   3/4 cup fresh or frozen blueberries

   2 tbsp ground flax seed

C: blueberries **P:** cottage cheese **F:** toasted almonds

- Place cottage cheese in a blender and blend until smooth.
- Remove and add pudding and vanilla.
- Place in a bowl and top with blueberries and sprinkle with ground flax seed and graham cracker crumbs.

Chocolate Almond Butter Treat

This is a perfect one to satisfy those late night cravings!

Prep Time: 5 mins
Cook Time: 10-15 mins
Serves 1

1/2 cup cottage cheese

1-2 tsp fat free vanilla pudding

1 tsp vanilla

1 whole wheat, sprouted grain or rice wrap

1 tbsp almond butter

a few dark chocolate chips

C: wrap **P:** cottage cheese **F:** almond butter

- Preheat oven to 350 degrees F.
- Blend cottage cheese in a blender.
- Stir in pudding and vanilla and set aside.
- Take your wrap and spread almond butter on half.
- Top with chocolate chips.
- Fold over and bake five to seven minutes until chips are melted and wrap is toasted.
- Cut your wrap into wedges and dip them into your vanilla sauce.

266

Strawberry Pudding Topped with Toasted Almonds & Chocolate Chips

Turn this into an indulgent dish by serving in a wine glass. You can also top with a few chocolate chips and a dollop of whipped cream for a real treat on those late night snack attacks!

Prep Time: 8 mins
Cook Time: 5 mins
Serves 1

3/4 cup yogurt
1-2 tbsp fat free vanilla pudding
5-8 strawberries
1-2 tbsp almonds, chopped or slivered
1 scoop protein powder
1 tbsp dark chocolate chips

C: strawberries **P:** protein powder/yogurt **F:** almonds

- Spread almonds in a single layer on a baking sheet and toast in the oven until golden brown.
- Mix yogurt, protein powder and pudding together. Top with strawberries and toasted almonds.

Yogurt Topped with Apples, Grapes and Toasted Walnuts

There is something about the combination of grapes, apples and walnuts. This is a great one for the kids to do as well.

Prep Time: 5 mins
Cook Time: 0 mins
Serves 1

3/4 cup of low fat yogurt
1 scoop, protein powder
1/2 apple sliced
8 grapes
1 tbsp toasted walnuts
a dash of cinnamon

C: yogurt, apple and grapes **P:** yogurt and protein powder **F:** walnuts

- Mix protein and yogurt. Top with chopped apples, grapes and walnuts.

Protein Vanilla Yogurt Crunch

This might be under treats, but it is also a quick and easy breakfast!

Prep Time: 10 mins
Cook Time: 0 mins
Serves 1

3/4 cup low fat yogurt
1 scoop protein powder
1 tbsp fat free vanilla pudding
1 tbsp whole grain cereal-any of your favourites
1 tbsp slivered almonds

C: cereal and yogurt **P:** protein powder **F:** cereal

- Mix yogurt, protein powder and pudding. Top with your favourite whole grain crunchy cereal.

Hemp Flaxseed Popcorn

Who doesn't like popcorn? This is a great treat for a Saturday night.

Prep Time: 0 mins
Cook Time: 5 mins

Serves 2

8 cups air popped popcorn

Topping:
1/4 cup hemp protein powder
1 tbsp flaxseed oil
sea salt to taste

- Mix protein powder, flaxseed oil and sea salt.
- Sprinkle over popcorn and enjoy.

KIDS' FAVOURITE RECIPES

Here are some of my daughter's favourite meal ideas. Yes, they're some of my favourites too - who doesn't like being a kid sometimes?

BREAKFAST
Dunkin' Pancake Fingers

Dunkin' Pancake Fingers allow children to play with their food - what child doesn't like that?

- Prepare the Blueberry Hazelnut Pancakes from page 245.
- Cut your pancakes into strips.
- Dunk into yogurt, applesauce, your favourite berry sauce or even a chocolate. butter mix (1 tsp cocoa, 1 tbsp peanut butter and a little milk to change the consistency).

Banana Split Breakfast Parfait

This may look fancy, but looks can be deceiving! It will take you no time at all and your children will feel like they're eating dessert for breakfast. You can even have your children make this one for you!

Prep Time: 5 mins
Cook Time: 0 mins
Serves 3

1 small banana
3 strawberries
1/4 cup blueberries
1/4 cup raspberries
1/4 cup oats
1/2 cup yogurt (your children's favourite)

Candied nuts:
1/4 cup mixed nuts
1 tsp honey
dash vanilla
sprinkle of cinnamon

C: fruit, oats **F:** nuts

- Place nuts, honey, vanilla and cinnamon in a non-stick pan, on low heat, stir to coat, toast until nuts are golden brown.
- Take the banana and slice it down the middle.
- Place banana slices on either side of a cup.
- Get creative and alternate the remaining ingredients.
- Top with the candied nuts.
- This is great to share.

Strawberry Oat Sundae

Your children will never know that this is healthy!

1 cup yogurt (any kind will do)
1/2 cup oats
1/2 - 1 cup fresh strawberries, sliced
1 tbsp candied nuts (see banana split breakfast parfait)

C: oats/strawberries **P:** yogurt **F:** nuts

- If you don't have a sundae-serving dish, then use one of your glasses.
- Layer yogurt, oats and strawberries until done.
- Top with dollop of yogurt, sprinkle with your candied nuts and enjoy!

LUNCH
Spider Caesar Chicken Wrap

A healthy lunch with a fun name!

Prep Time: 10 mins
cook time: 0 mins
serves 1

1/2 boneless chicken breast, cooked
1 whole wheat /sprouted grain or rice wrap
1 tbsp of parmesan cheese
1 tbsp of low-fat caesar dressing
8 thin slices of your child's favourite veggies (carrots, celery, cucumber)
tomatoes and onions if your child likes it

C: wrap **P:** chicken **F:** Cheese

- Place chicken, parmesan cheese, low-fat caesar dressing in a wrap and roll it up.
- Take your eight thinly sliced veggies and press them it to the sides of the wrap to make the legs.
- Cut a cherry tomato in half for the eyes.

Banana Flower Dip

Your child will love to receive flowers - especially for lunch! This is easy for kids to make too.

Prep Time: 10 mins
Cook Time: 0 mins
Serves 1

1 banana
1 whole wheat, sprouted grain or rice wrap
2 tbsp peanut, almond or cashew butter
3 sliced strawberries
1/2 cup yogurt, any flavour
1 celery stick

C: wrap **P:** yogurt and peanut butter **F:** peanut butter

- Place wrap flat on the counter.
- Spread peanut butter and place the banana in the middle.
- Roll up and slice into one inch rounds.
- On a pretty plate, place the wrap slices in a circle (this is the start of the flower).
- Add some colour by placing the strawberry slices in between every second wrap slice.
- Place the celery stick as the stem.
- Serve with a side of yogurt for dipping.

Veggies and Hummus

These are a great snack but also a great way to have the veggies go down. Make a double batch and keep it handy in your fridge for when you need something quick!

Prep Time: 10-15 mins
Cook Time: 0 mins
Serves 4

    1 can chickpeas

    3 garlic cloves

    2 tbsp tahini paste

    1 tsp lemon juice

    4 cups sliced veggies

    3-4 whole wheat pita cut into triangles

C: chickpeas **P:** chickpeas **F:** tahini paste

- Place all in a blender until smooth and serve with your favourite veggies and pita pieces.

DINNER
Chicken Fingers and Fries in a Bag

Trust me when I say it's all about the looks. This is a quick and simple meal and your kids will think and feel as if they are in a restaurant! The chicken fingers are also great to freeze for a Ticket Meal.

Prep Time: 20 mins
Cook Time: 35 mins
Serves 4

4 boneless chicken breasts
2 large yams
1/2 cup Italian low fat, low sodium dressing
1/4 cup parmesan cheese

Coating:
1 cup oats
1/3 cup ground flax seeds
1 tsp garlic powder

C: yams or potatoes **P:** chicken **F:** parmesan cheese

Chicken Fingers:
- Cut chicken breasts into strips (it's easier if it's a little frozen in the middle).
- Mix coating mixture together.
- Coat chicken with Italian dressing and then coating mixture.
- Place in a non-stick frying pan and place in the oven 375 degrees F. or grill, they turn out crispier in a non-stick frying pan.
- Cook for 10 minutes then flip to the other side for another 10-15 minutes.

Yam Fries:
- Preheat oven to 375 degrees F.
- Cut yams into wedges.
- Coat in salad dressing (use a different container then previously used) and place on a non-stick cookie sheet.
- Sprinkle with parmesan cheese.
- Bake in the oven for 30-35 minutes, turning every 15 minutes.

- Write your child's name on a brown paper bag and even a little message or a topic of conversation for dinner time. Toss the chicken fingers and fries into the bag, lined with a little wax paper, and serve.

Bowtie Rainbow Chicken

Prep Time: 10 mins
Cook Time: 20 mins
Serves 4

2 cups whole wheat noodles (or any other shape that your child likes)
4 boneless chicken breasts
1-2 cups of broccoli (fresh or frozen)
10-12 cherry tomatoes, halved
1/2 cup onion, chopped
1-2 garlic cloves
1-2 tbsp canola oil
1/4 cup chicken broth
1/4 parmesan cheese

C: pasta **P:** chicken **F:** parmesan cheese and canola oil

- Cook noodles as per package instructions.
- In a non stick frying pan heat canola oil.
- Sauté garlic and onions until onions are translucent.
- Add chicken, when chicken is partially cooked add broccoli, cook for another ten minutes.
- Once chicken and broccoli are cooked.
- Add cooked bowtie noodles and chicken broth, and halved cherry tomatoes, stir and heat through.
- Serve topped with parmesan cheese and a side salad.

Taco Cups

Your children will think you are totally a top chef in the kitchen - little do they know how quick and easy they really are!

Prep Time: 25 mins
Cook Time: 15 mins
Serves 4

1 lb lean ground beef
1 small onion
1 package low sodium taco seasoning
1/2 cup low fat cheddar cheese
8 small whole grain, sprouted grain or rice tortilla shells
1 small tomato, diced
5 green onions
1 cup salsa
1/2 cup yogurt cheese (or fat free sour cream or even blended cottage cheese if you like)
iceberg lettuce, chopped

C: tortilla shells **P:** ground beef **F:** ground beef, sour cream, cheese

Taco cups:
- Preheat oven to 375 F.
- Place shell in a non-stick muffin tin and carefully fold edges in.
- Bake for 5-7 minutes until edges are brown.

Meat:
- Sauté onion and ground beef in a non-stick frying pan.
- Once browned, add taco seasoning. Following directions on seasoning packet.
- Place meat mixture in the bottom of the taco cups.
- Have fun with the remainder of the ingredients by filling the cup to the top!

Meatball Boats

Don't be fooled by the name, these are just as good for the parents!

Prep Time: 15 mins
Cook Time: 35 mins
Serves 4

1 lb extra lean ground beef

1-2 garlic cloves

1 small onion

3 tbsp ground flaxseed

2 egg whites

1/2 tsp garlic powder

3 tsp italian herbs

1 jar spaghetti sauce

1/2 cup rolled oats

2 whole wheat pitas

2-4 tbsp parmesan cheese

C: pita **P:** beef **F:** parmesan cheese

- Preheat oven to 350 F.
- Mix first seven ingredients in a large bowl.
- Roll into 1" balls and coat with oats.
- Bake in oven for 30-35 minutes until golden brown.
- Cover with sauce and bake for another 5 minutes.
- Place in pitas and top with parmesan cheese.
- Serve with a side salad.

SNACKS
Fruit Kabobs with Yogurt Dip

Prep Time: 4 mins
Cook Time: 0 mins
Serves 1

1/2 cantaloupe
1/2 cup grapes
4 strawberries
1 tangerine or orange

- Wash and cut fruit into bite size shapes (a melon baller works best for melons).
- Place on wooden skewers in a color pattern alternating with each fruit.
- Serve with your child's favourite yogurt.

Spiced Apple Cups

These are quick and easy and great to serve as dessert or an afternoon treat. This is also something you can get your kids to do while you prep for dinner.

Prep Time: 10 mins
Cook Time: 25 mins
Serves 4

4 small apples peeled and sliced
1-2 cups low fat yogurt or cottage cheese
1/2 cup walnuts

Topping:
3/4 cup oats
1/2 cup brown sugar, honey or agave nectar or other sweetener
3 tbsp ground flax seeds
1 tsp cinnamon

C: apples **P:** yogurt cottage cheese **F:** walnuts

- Preheat oven to 350 degrees F.
- Line muffin tin with liners.
- Place apple slices evenly in each muffin tin.
- Mix, oats, brown sugar, honey or agave nectar or other sweetener, ground flax seeds, and cinnamon together.
- Cover apples with topping mixture.
- Top with nuts and bake for 25-30 minutes.
- Serve with a dollop of low fat yogurt or blended cottage cheese.

Frozen Almond Butter Surprise

This one is great, and your children will have fun eating it too!

Prep Time: 20 mins
Cook Time: 15 mins
Serves 4

2 cups of your child's favourite yogurt

2 tbsp almond butter or peanut butter

2-4 tbsp fat-free chocolate pudding mix

12 surprises: fresh fruit, cookie pieces, M&Ms and so forth

C: yogurt **P:** yogurt **F:** almond butter

- Mix the first three ingredients together and set aside.
- Line a small muffin tin with liners and place the surprise at the bottom (silicone liners work best).
- Fill a cookie press with yogurt mixture.
- Cover each surprise with yogurt mixture and place in the freezer until frozen (about 30-60 minutes).
- Remove from freezer and place in a freezer-safe bag for storage.
- I like to use different coloured muffin liners and coordinate them so I remember which surprise is in which colour.

Index

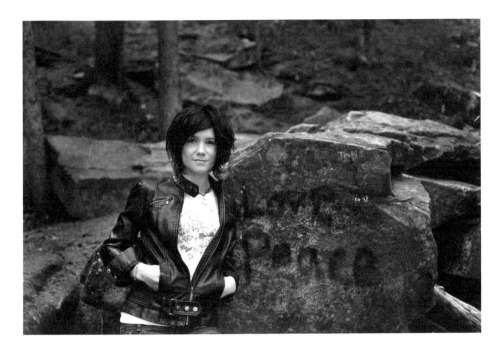

ABOUT THE AUTHOR

Sean Liv – Fitness Expert, Life Strategist and Motivational Speaker

Sean Liv struggled for years with physical abuse, drug abuse and her weight. After losing 90 pounds and overcoming addictions, depression and negativity, she was amazed at the freedom she finally felt. She works with clients to show them how to ignite their own inner power.

The name "Liv" comes from a combination of life, inspiration and vitality – three things that are central to Sean's life and philosophy.

Sean designed the The Ticket to Change Challenge to help people understand the holistic link between a healthy body, a healthy spirit and a healthy mind. With Sean's guidance and experience, participants in the Challenge are active participants, finding their own journey to complete wellness. They learn how to tap into their limitless potential, transforming their bodies, minds and spirits to live the life of their dreams.

If you'd like to participate in "**The Ticket to Change**", a 13-week transformational challenge – visit our website to find challenge dates near you:

www.thetickettochange.com

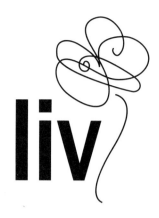

LIV IS AN INVITATION TO A NEW WAY OF LIVING.

Realize you have the POWER! The power of courage, the power of voice, the power in your life!

Life: Uncover your meaning of life, then with courage, strength and faith, release, forgive and accept. You will then be in the present moment and aligned in the direction of your desires.

Inspiration: Allow your desires to become your REAL Motivation - see who you truly are, and who you deserve to become. When you are motivated, you are able to inspire.

Vitality: Find the love of life! Be present in your vitality. Be joyful and courageous. Chart the path to the life you've always wanted.

The choice is yours. Will you accept this invitation to LIV?